BATTLE IN MY WOMB

The story of a country(the pregnant sickle cell warrior) in world war II. Did the country survive?

DR. AGBOOLA EMMANUEL

CHAPTER 1 1
BOOK ENDORSEMENT: 2
CHAPTER 2 8
THE 3 YEARS WAR 8
    THE PREGNANT SICKLE CELL PATIENT (9 MONTHS PREGNANCY, 3 MONTHS PRE-CONCEPTUAL CARE, 6 WEEKS PUERPERIUM, 2 YEARS BREASTFEEDING) 8
    SO HOW DID THE OPPOSITION MILITARIES AND COUNTRIES GET TO KNOW ABOUT THE NEW BILL THAT WAS MADE INTO THE LAW? 35
    THE BATTLE: 37
    THE LABOUR(CHILD BIRTH) 45
    NOT ALL STUDENTS MADE IT TO THE NINTH MONTH 50
    LABOUR CONTINUES 59
CHAPTER 3 68
ACADEMIC ASPECT OF THIS BOOK 68
    The sickle cell girl child 68
    THE MANAGEMENT OF MENSTRUAL PAIN THAT COMES WITH MENSTRUAL FLOW AND WHICH TRIGGERS SC CRISIS 69
    THE PRECONCEPTUAL CARE 69
    ANTENATAL CARE 75

MANAGING OTHER COMPLICATIONS OF SICKLE DURING ANTENATAL CARE..................................87

INTRAPARTUM CARE..93

POSTPARTUM CARE.. 96

CHAPTER 4.. 103

BONUSES:... 103

1. NAIRA MARLEY AND MOHBAD SAGA :..........104

2. THE CURE TO SICKLE CELL DISEASE: BONE MARROW TRANSPLANT!...................................... 113

SICKLE CELL AND THE GOSPEL; ANY RELATIONSHIP?..113

3. ISRAEL AND PALESTINE are not the only locations where there are bomb blasts... 118

4. ATIKU ABUBAKAR'S state (Adamawa, Nigeria), there lived a farmer, who was very rich, but not so intelligent...122

5. EMERGENCY!...125

6. SICKLE CELL CHILD CARE..................................128

7. DEPRESSION IS COMMON AMONG SICKLE CELL PATIENTS...132

PSYCHOTHERAPY TIPS AND OTHER MEASURES FOR SICKLE CELL PATIENTS..................................132

8. PREGNANT SICKLE CELL PATIENT...................147

9. WASTED LIFE CAUSED BY CARELESSNESS BEFORE, DURING AND AFTER PREGNANCY; DAMAGE COULD BE IRREVERSIBLE AND COULD COST YOU MORE THAN $1,000,000!......................154

CHAPTER 1

BOOK ENDORSEMENT:

Martin Luther King Jr [till date] is one of the United States citizens who won a NOBEL PRIZE.

Like other NOBEL PRIZE winners, he is known as a NOBEL LAUREATE.

A Laureate is a person who is honoured with an award for outstanding
CREATIVE OR INTELLECTUAL ACHIEVEMENT.

Professor Adeyinka Falusi Gladys(Nigeria) is another LAUREATE who won something synonymous with a NOBEL PRIZE.

She became a LAUREATE in 2001 after her novel discovery in hereditary blood diseases [SICKLE CELL DISEASE AND ALPHA THALASSEMIA].

The award won is known as the L'Oréal-UNESCO Awards for Women in Sciences.

Reference:

https://www.fondationloreal.com/our-programs-women-science/laureates-loreal-unesco-women-science-international-award

Professor Adeyinka Falusi PhD, (FAS, FAMedS, NPOM, L'Oreal UNESCO Laureate Africa), has this to say about my books.

Before I tell you what she says, I'll like to say it's a big deal that I have a request from this internationally recognised woman Adeyinka Falusi (who has a novel discovery in Haematology); to co-author her book with her, among other dignitaries, (because of the simplicity of my books for the understanding of the layman).

Because of my association with her, I now have an association (directly or indirectly) with LAUREL UNESCO!

Read carefully what she has to say about my books:

"MY ENDORSEMENT OF DR AGBOOLA'S BOOKS

These books are:

• SHINING THROUGH THE DARK TUNNEL

• SICKLE CELL UNMASKED

What stands out for me as the most remarkable and unforgettable moment reading through these books and his other writings can be briefly described below as:

The emotionally laden autobiography of his life is truly remarkable.

Through about 24 complications including Suicide, OCD, PTSD, Tuberculosis and about 100 hospitalizations, verbal and direct abuses and even absenteeism and denial of University Admissions that were beyond his control, he was able to comport himself and remain focused.

I am taken in by his honesty of purpose where he described why the non-affected people in the society should flee from the much-dreaded Sickle Cell Disease in their families.

This is really commendable as most People Living with Sickle Cell Disease (PLWSCD) will not speak in this manner.

A majority would be so partisan about themselves to claim that they do not suffer any setbacks by this disease or that the challenges experienced are being magnified.

Some even express that the disease is a blessing in their lives. Dr Agboola, on the other hand, has come out in a more truthful manner and has shown vividly what this disease has cost him but that nonetheless, his courage has seen him through it all.

The medical expertise of Dr Agboola brings to the fore a wealth of knowledge through his Educational teachings and commendable gentle persuation to learning the simple rudiments of Sickle Cell Disease including Education, and management of the Disease.

These incorporate the Paediatrics, Psychiatric, Gynacological, Obstetrics details with the simplest approach possible.

His spiritual acumen in bringing the details of these medical issues to everyone, For example, where he uses biblical context to illustrate Blood Transfusion and Bone Marrow Transplantation in his latest writings, this spiritual approach, endears a large proportion of the population to him as Nigeria is a spiritually tilted community.

Not only this, unlike most books published globally, Dr Agboola in his books has brought out his message in the simplest layman's language that anyone at least with a high school background can relate with to understand his presentations.

What gets one thinking about the author is the survival instinct and tenacity of purpose of this 31-year-old learned Warrior- Dr Agboola.

His Education as a Medical Doctor has been appropriately called to use in the way he has linked his experience to his daily activities and challenges.

I cannot but label Dr Agboola as a brave, determined, focused, hardworking, brilliant diligent and prayerful Warrior who makes the most of each day the Almighty God has given him to live.

I am really impressed, and I always feel committed to help him in any way I possibly can as an advocate of People Living With Sickle Cell Disease (PLWSCD).

I have learnt through my 40 years of exposure on the bench and in the field, the theoretical and practical challenges of Sickle Cell Disorder firsthand.

Kudos to Dr Agboola for his efforts again.

He is indeed an asset to his family, People Living With Sickle Cell Disease (PLWSCD), the Nigerian and Global Community.

He continues to bridge the gap between Patients and Professionals bringing new insights and understanding to the psycho-social inner beings of the People Living With Sickle Cell Disease (PLWSCD) globally.

I am privileged as an advocate to comment on these books and recommend them for reading by all in Nigeria- a country which carries the highest burden of Sickle Cell Disease globally.

With very best wishes.

PROFESSOR ADEYINKA FALUSI GLADYS

•PhD

•FAS [Fellow of the Nigerian Academy of Science]

•FAMedS

•NPOM [National Productivity Order of Merit Award]

•L'Oreal UNESCO Laureate Africa And The Arab States."

"I need say no more"

Kindly place your orders for each book now (hardcopies or soft copies), through the links below :

https://www.amazon.com/dp/B0C7LHCGB9

https://www.amazon.com/dp/B0C3SVCSVC

WHY SHOULD YOU LISTEN TO ME?

I have spent approximately 6 years practising in the medical and dental profession.

I'll clock 6 years on 12th April 2024.

On 26th January 2018[more than 6 years ago], I bagged my degree in dental surgery from the **FIRST AND THE BEST** University in Nigeria-University of Ibadan!

On the 12th of April 2018, in the University College Hospital (The **FIRST TEACHING HOSPITAL IN NIGERIA**), I got inducted into the Medical and Dental Profession.

In 2018 I got an offer for my Housemanship in the same institution (University College Hospital), **BUT I DECLINED IT!**

31st December 2021, I got a job with the Federal Medical Centre Makurdi, Benue State Nigeria;

I have spent more than *2 YEARS PRACTISING AS A DENTAL SURGEON IN THIS FEDERAL GOVERNMENT INSTITUTION!*

Also, *I'll soon relocate to the United Kingdom* for a job opportunity as a dental surgeon *or to the United States for my postgraduate program*.

I have received several awards before and after my undergraduate years.

The ones I got in high school were academic awards.

One of them is the International Junior Science Olympiad Oyo State Finalist award(October 2006).

The others are best student awards, received in 5 different subjects in highschool.

I also took a research-related course conducted by the Collaborative Institutional Training Initiative in 2020,

(Good Clinical Practice Course
under requirements set by the West African Bioethics Training Program).

My patients love me so much because of my empathy and how I'm able to relate with their symptoms, especially toothaches.

Many of my patients are also wowed at how my professionalism and "babyface" (young looks) could meet in just one body!

Many of them are also amused & amazed by, and feel relaxed and safe with my unique feminine voice!

In all these achievements and qualities, I have unbelievably surmounted approximately 26 complications and comorbidities of sickle cell anaemia within a timeframe of 32 years [just like the professor I quoted mentioned].

I have put my experience [both as a patient living with sickle cell disease, and as a doctor who has studied the nitty-gritty of managing the disease],

in two beautiful and highly impactful books titled, **"SHINING THROUGH THE DARK TUNNEL"** and **"SICKLE CELL UNMASKED"**.

I'm certain that you are interested in getting these books on sickle cell disease.

Kindly get them through the links below:

https://www.amazon.com/dp/B0C7LHCGB9

https://www.amazon.com/dp/B0C3SVCSVC

WHAT ARE THE AUTHORITIES IN THE MEDICAL PROFESSION AND OTHER PEOPLE SAYING ABOUT MY FIRST TWO BOOKS ON SICKLE CELL DISEASE?

This simplified explanation of sickle cell anaemia is really wholesome and down to earth. It's so simple everyone can understand sickle cell ailments without a university education. Thanks to Dr Agboola for this welcome job.

Dr. N. B. Ola (Consultant Anaesthetist and Founder of Chrisbo hb champions club:sickle cell support foundation.
)

Dr Agboola has put in a great deal of effort in making otherwise complex medical subjects appear so simple in layman's terms. The turbulent journey of that little, almost imperceptible alteration in the genetic makeup which led to myriads of systemic manifestations (symptoms and signs) and complications of sickle cell disease were laid bare. He used allegories to weave in difficult topics, cutting off jargons to reach the kernel of the matter.

This book explains sickle cell disease in an animating manner, making the readers empathetic to the pains of the warriors.

Dr Akunwata Chima

Consultant Haematologist

University College Hospital, Ibadan.

Let me commend the author who is himself a SCA warrior for painstakingly explaining in simple terms the genetic basis for the origin of Sickle Cell Anaemia as well as the series of events that eventually lead to the clinical manifestation of the disease. The use of beautiful analogies will definitely help those who may read this book to understand Sickle Cell Anaemia better.

I therefore recommend this book to all warriors, caregivers and the general public.

Dr. Aondover Mke

Senior Registrar Haematology Dept

(Benue State University Teaching Hospital)

This book has been a fun read. The balance between humour and seriousness is perfect. The stories have made it simple for the layman. Any simpler and it would have been " ABC OF SICKLE CELL FOR DUMMIES." Most important to note is that the writer has experienced and is still experiencing the ups and downs of sickle cell anaemia.

Doctor Alexander Abu (Consultant, Pathologist, Federal Medical Centre, Makurdi)

Dr. Agboola's book is an encyclopaedia of life with sickle cell, simplified for the layman. It is a fascinating book filled with insights from a sickle cell warrior-medical doctor

AyoOla OlaJide

Editor, Sickle Cell News

Author, Menace In My Blood - my affliction with sickle cell anaemia

President, Ikorodu Sickle Cell Club

Sickle cell is a group of inherited red blood cell disorder, the red cell becomes hard and sticky and looks like a C shape farm tool called a sickle.

Haemoglobin electrophoresis is the gold standard method for diagnosis of Haemoglobin genotype which each individual is supposed to undergo at early stage of their lives and a must do for intending couples.

The writer of this book, Dr Emmanuel Agboola is a doctor, a sickle cell warrior and is well known to me. his personal experience as a sickle cell subject will teach us a lot of things and elucidate us on most of the complications of sickle cell.

I therefore recommend this book for individuals, families, hospitals and schools to have a copy in their library.

Swem Collins (MSc, FMLSCN, FAMLSN) Ag. HOD Haematology/ DDMLS FMC MAKURDI.

In this "masterpiece", the Author has presented an in-depth knowledge of Sickle Cell Disease (SCD) and explored The Truths and Myths of Living with the condition.

This Quintessential work embellished with tales/parables including personal experiences connecting nature and nurture, also involving other fields of human endeavour (Agriculture, Engineering, Architecture and Artisans) not solely Medicine, is concisely packaged to enable all and sundry have a simplistic information on the topic.

Sicklers, their family members/relatives and friends, their managers (Medical Personnel) and indeed laymen and professionals will undoubtedly find this book as a suitable **Guide** to: Stemming-down the occurrence of the disease (Preventive); Giving succour to the sufferers and limiting their progression to complications/analgesic addiction (Curative); Finding fulfilment and attaining their **peak** despite the **burden** of the disease (Palliative).

Finally, trusting the power of the Divine Healer to sail them through.

Dr. Orimoloye Augustina O.

This book by Dr. Emmanuel Agboola is an incisive and breath-taking exploration into the world of sickle cell anaemia. The writer tells his real-life story in a captivating and engaging fashion. He is not an outsider looking in, but a sufferer himself. It becomes even more interesting that he is also a sufferer. The book not only tells us about the everyday and real-life travails of a sickle cell sufferer, but goes deeper to educate the general public on ways of avoiding this terribly debilitating and life-altering condition altogether. It is an indispensable guide that should be on every family's and every adult's bookshelf.

Barrister Chuks Okoronkwo, FIPMD

What stood out for me in this book was how Dr Emmanuel married real life experiences with the disordered physiological processes associated with Sickle cell disease so that the lay man could have an in-depth understanding of the disease condition.

Dr. Oluchi Nwankwo

This book, which is focused on sickle cell anaemia, reveals how medically wrong decisions can result in a lifetime painful and life-threatening condition; sickle cell anaemia. It depicts this, using stories in different areas of life.

The author, Dr Agboola Tobiloba, a highly gifted writer, does an excellent work in educating people on sickle cell anaemia and in discouraging reproduction that would result in the illness. It's a must read.

Dr. Oji Nnanyelugo M.

This is a masterpiece I feel every parent and intending couples should read. My close friend was going to make a grave mistake of getting married to someone who's AS like him. He cited different medical interventions they could undergo to ensure they don't have kids with sickle cell anaemia. I had to counsel him from my experience and examples from this book. Thank God he yielded though it was a tough call.

A very big thank you to the writer as this will go a long way in ending this mistake people make consciously and unconsciously.

Mr. Tobi

(Masters in Public Health University of Ibadan)

It is so informative and such a detailed explanation of Sickle Cell Disease. The value is more than the cost. I will say information is life, you need to get a copy.

Mr. Bolade

(Chartered Accountant and Sickle Cell Warrior)

Dr. Tobi's style of bringing the reality of sickle cell into a storyline that everyone can identify with, is laudable.

Most of us are scared and easily get bored with big medical terms, but in these books, he made it so simple, such that even young people can understand what he is talking about.

People hardly believe what we say, but nobody doubts your experience that they are aware of.

Emmanuel's experience of over thirty years, in his victorious fight of faith against sickle cell (by the way that's the only fight the scriptures permit us to fight), of which I have the privilege of being part of, now made available in print is a book I will like to recommend that you read, buy as a gift for anyone you know that is going through the challenge in their lives. It will serve as a guide from the medical perspective, and of course provide step by step instructions in your quest to experience the same thing, Dr. Tobi experienced.

Pastor Idowu Oluwarotimi

Ibadan, 2023.

Tobi's secondary school Geography teacher.

This book is a very powerful book that will encourage everyone to get it. It is not just for Sickle cell patients. It is a knowledge packed book. The author wrote the book in an intricate way that you will find every page intriguing

Ms Aanuoluwapo (A Psychology Undergraduate)

I really like this book. It's an eye opener. Especially the part where you explained the blood compatibility on blood group and genotype.

I really enjoyed the part where you explained the SS blood circulation using the farm as an illustration.

More wins to you sir.

Ms PECULIAR (MOTHER TO A SICKLE CELL WARRIOR)

Ingenious...

Thought-provoking and enlightening. Simply beautiful.

Mrs. Idowu (My Secondary School Teacher and Mother to a Sickle Cell Warrior)

CHAPTER 2

THE 3 YEARS WAR

THE PREGNANT SICKLE CELL PATIENT (9 MONTHS PREGNANCY, 3 MONTHS PRE-CONCEPTUAL CARE, 6 WEEKS PUERPERIUM, 2 YEARS BREASTFEEDING)

In 1900, there lived a country that was always attacked by war. The name of the country was Pregnickle.

Before this time, there were ancient geographical boundaries and barriers that protected this country from its invaders.(innate immunity)

These boundaries include hills, rocks, oceans(humoral innate immunity) and forests.

Like the natural boundaries of China which protects it from invaders, Pregnickle also has deserts, mountains(the skin, nasal hair and the mucosa) and seas(humoral innate immunity) around it.

Like Korah, Dathan and Abiram(in the bible) were swallowed up by the earth as they assaulted Moses, there were times when even the earthquake and volcanic eruptions would swallow up their invaders, alongside the bullet proofs they put on(spleen and phagocytosis).

They even built abysses(pits) during wars where some of the opposition armies fell into(spleen and phagocytosis).

Like the "indomitable" walls of Jericho, this country also has heavily built walls around it, for security purposes.

Some of the natives of Pregnickle were born natural fighters(natural killer cells).

They also trained lions, hyenas, tigers, wolves and foxes which helped to defeat soldiers that wore breastplates, helmets and bullet proofs(phagocytosis of encapsulated organisms).

As Pregnickle advanced in civilisation, it trained military personnels who fought on the land(the army), in the seas and other water bodies(the marine corps, submarines, the navy and the coast guard); and in the air(the air force and the space force).

AmunistatA is a notable Force to reckon with in the training of Pregnickle's military and in the evolution of a civilised and sophisticated military force in Pregnickle!

Pregnickle had 5 warships, 11 aircraft carriers/super carriers, 15,000 operational & military aircrafts, 406 massive stock pile of intercontinental ballistic missiles[ICBMS](both conventional and nuclear) and 170 military satellites.

The Submarine of Pregnickle also has Submarine-launched Ballistic Missiles[SLBMS].

The LGM-30 MINUTEMAN III is one of the land based ICBMS developed by AmunistatA for Pregnickle.

On behalf of Pregnickle, AmunistatA in the course of 5 decades upgraded and refurbished these arsenals and fire powers [the ICBMS].

The upgrade program spanned across the rocket propulsion engines, the propellants used, the guidance system and finally to the flight control services!

The newest version of these ICBMS can travel for as far as 8,000 miles; a distance greater than 7,917.5 miles[the diameter of the world!].

This version can carry up to 330 kilotons of nuclear warheads.

These warheads are capable of being targeted to different locations and entirely in different directions with a technology known as MULTIPLE INDEPENDENTLY TARGETABLE REENTRY VEHICLE[MIRV].

AmunistatA also advanced the military of Pregnickle in technology and precision by developing smart bombs also known as PRECISION-GUIDED MUNITIONS [PGMs].

These have highly precise accuracy in hitting targets and they cause very little or minimal collateral damages; they are extremely efficient and effective!

Experimental comparisons show that non-guided missiles (91% of all missiles shot] accounted for just 25% of successful hits; while PGMs[9% of all missiles shot] accounted for a whopping 75% successful hits!

Very interesting, right?

These PGMs use technologies such as the GLOBAL POSITIONING SYSTEM or GPS of satellites to achieve precise hits.

Because some parts of the world where the enemies of Pregnickle are, do not have a reliably available GPS and because the weather conditions sometimes do not favour this technology,

the AmunistatA Office of the Naval Research[AONR], AmunistatA Naval Surface Warfare Centre[ANSWC], and the AmunistatA Army Research Laboratories[AARL] have all collaborated on behalf of Pregnickle to develop

ARTILLERY SMART NEW MACHINES that don't need GPS for their precision hits!

That's the first of its kind in the history of man!

The project is known as MOVING TARGET ARTILLERY ROUNDS[MTAR]!

It is good to note that all branches of the military of Pregnickle[the navy, the airforce and the army] use the IBMs, the PGMs and the MTAR.

The M777A2 [one of the two types of M777 HOWITZER that Pregnickle has] uses a digital fire-control system similar to that found on self-propelled howitzers [such as the M109A6].

The novelle MTAR shells can surprisingly be fired from this pre-existing M777A2 155mm towed howitzer and the M109A7 integrated management self-propelled 155mm artillery systems already in use by Pregnickle's military!

With the use of rocket boosters to propel these MTAR shells, they can travel for as far as 40 to 60 miles; an excellent feature I think!

AmunistatA also blessed the airforce of Pregnickle with a thousand UNMANNED COMBAT AERIAL VEHICLES (UCAV), also known as COMBAT DRONES and colloquially shortened as DRONES or BATTLEFIELD UAVs.

For a layman like you, you may like to stick with the term "DRONES".

Drones for several decades have functioned primarily in prominent surveillance missions of the army of Pregnickle.

After a brutal attack however which almost wiped out the entire country, drones were rapidly weaponised i.e. they could now function like the fighter jets.

They could now function as offensive weapons.

The most advanced and sophisticated of the drones used in the air force and military of Pregnickle include the LOCKHEED MARTIN RQ-170 SENTINEL and BOEING MQ-25 STINGRAY.

They are noted for both their sophisticated surveillance prowess and attack precision and accuracy.

Other reconnaissance (surveillance) aircrafts that were developed by AmunistatA for Pregnickle in the past include:

the LOCKHEED SR-71 "BLACKBIRD", a long-range, high-altitude, mach 3+ STRATEGIC RECONNAISSANCE AIRCRAFT,

and its predecessor, LOCKHEED A-12 (also a STRATEGIC RECONNAISSANCE AIRCRAFT)!

Of the 13,209 aircrafts in Pregnickle, there were 3000 stealth aircrafts designed to deliver assignments of "silent killings".

Some of the stealth aircrafts include AIR SUPERIORITY FIGHTERS like F-22 RAPTOR, F-35 JOINT STRIKE FIGHTER and HEAVY BOMBERS like the B-2 SPIRIT, F-117 NIGHTHAWK stealth attack aircraft.

Others include CHENGDU J-20 AND SUKHOI SU-57.

These stealth aircrafts cannot be detected by the radar defence system of most countries!

Fighter jets constitute the fleet of Pregnickle's air force as well!

There are about 1,854 fighter aircrafts, 896 attack aircrafts, 2,648 trainers, 695 special mission aircrafts, 606 tanker fleet, 1,000 attack helicopters, 5,737 helicopters and 957 transport aircrafts in Pregnickle!

The fighter jets and helicopters are a force to reckon with in the air force of Pregnickle!

As mentioned earlier, one of the functions of the air force of Pregnickle is to go on reconnaissance or surveillance missions.

The navy of Pregnickle has about 75 destroyers on the seas.

One of the navy's missions and assignments include attacking pirates, supporting and collaborating with the Airforce.

In the deep seas, Pregnickle's navy could spend close to 2 years away from the land and their families.

Their saving grace is the availability of good food and diets made available by the chefs in the fleet.

There were grocery stores, games and sport complexes, and many other things that made the troops feel less away from home!

Supplies to the stores and the kitchens come from the land and it is mandatory that the aircraft carriers do not run out of supply.

Their supplies are usually brought by cargo aircrafts.

Aircraft carriers are synonymous to Noah's ark where it's another life entirely.

The aircraft carriers have an exceedingly spacious landing space from which aircrafts can equally take off; simply put, an airport!

The sleeping conditions and comfort however are not usually perfect in an aircraft carrier!

The name of the 11 aircraft carriers that Pregnickle has is the NUCLEAR-POWERED NIMITZ CLASS AIRCRAFT CARRIER!

The Nimitz Class aircraft carriers each can carry up to 70 aircrafts at a time.

Pregnickle also had armoured tanks(6,300 in number) and other armoured vehicles which were used in the frontlines of the battlefield.

These were used by the land troops (the army).

Some of these armoured vehicles were named earlier: the M777A2 [one of the two types of M777 HOWITZER] and the M109A6.

One of the missions and assignments of the army include rescuing hostages.

They were also trained in physical combat and demolition assignments.

Some of the training underwent by some of the military personnels forbid them to take alcohol or any psychoactive substance.

Some of them, for their kind of assignments, do not live with the civilians.

This is particularly common with military squads assigned to very secretive and high profile assignments.

The land troop (army) of Pregnickle, altogether has 1,595 self-propelled artillery, 2,800 towed artillery and 1,410 rocket projectors.

The armoured tanks remain the most valuable assets of the land troops (the army).

They include the M1A2 ABRAMS, the most powerful armoured tanks!

The other assets with which the Navy of Pregnickle was equipped include 64 submarines, 9 helicopter carriers, 8 mine warfare ships, 5 Patrol ships and 23 Corvettes!

Together with the aircraft carriers, the surface and underwater vessels(guided missile cruisers, a destroyer squadron, attack submarines, and other support vessels) form THE CARRIER STRIKE GROUPS of Pregnickle's navy.

There were 9 powerful carrier strike groups in the navy of Pregnickle!

The carrier strike groups are an intelligently organised sea or ocean warfare team designed to attack the enemies and defend [the massive aircraft carriers and its inhabitants especially].

Apart from the Nimitz Class aircraft carriers, AmunistatA developed another set of 11 aircraft carriers that were superior in technological advancement to the Nimitz Class.

AmunistatA did this after two decades of the existence of the Nimitz Class.

The name of these carriers is the GERALD R FORD-CLASS.

Pregnickle also had nuclear weapons which include about 5,428 nuclear warheads.

Some of the trainings the military students of Pregnickle underwent include:

Sprinting 200 metres with a load of 70 pounds on their backs!

Diving into the deep blue cold sea(the navy).

Trust shots(allowing a colleague to point a gun at you; synonymous with a firing squad, in an attempt to shoot your bullet-proofed chest).

White noise(a phase where potential recruits are kept in a room devoid of sound and light; research makes it clear that this is a form of psychological torture for which the person inflicting it can be sued. It's against human rights!)

Performing surgeries on self.

Pain, prick, itch, sting and bite endurance.

The students in the navy of Pregnickle have a four week intensive training called hell week!

The students in the hell week are constantly in motion;

running,

swimming,

paddling,

carrying heavy rubber boats on their heads,

doing log physical training (carrying heavy logs of wood as a team),

sit-ups,

push-ups,

rolling in the sand,

slogging through the mud,

paddling boats and

doing surf passage(riding the boats against the waves)

During the hell week, the potential recruits are wet, cold and sandy!

Most of the training especially those of hell week were meant to break the wills of these potential recruits!

Throughout the 4 week long hell week, potential recruits would be deprived of sleep and food!

During hell week, potential recruits of Pregnickle's navy were immersed in $45°$ F cold water for 90 minutes.

Most of them reach the exhaustion/ subconsciousness stage after about a half an hour in water of 40–50° F.

Their training was conducted in the seas off the coasts of Southern California and Mid-Atlantic.

Most of them would be unable to answer simple questions, develop slurring of speech, exhibit lack of attention, and are incapable of doing simple tasks!

These draw extreme scrutiny from trainers.

Anyone showing signs of hypothermia or extreme mental or physical fatigue aren't allowed to continue with the hell week training.

They drop out of this training! [spontaneous abortion, stillbirth]

An average Pregnickle navy personnel that survives hell week can hold his breath for 2-3 minutes during underwater exercises, but with proper training, some can extend it to 5 minutes or more.

The training is that brutal!

Asides hell week and trust shots, the torture to test for loyalty is one of the very final phases of the training in the military of Pregnickle.

The potential recruits undergo several tortures meant to break them physically and mentally.

These torture include white noise, electrocution, torture with an electric fiery hot pressing iron, amputation of fingers, toes and limbs, beating with strokes laden with sharps, crowning their heads with thorns like those of Jesus, sprinkling salt and pepper on wounds and injured areas, plucking/ cutting off of ears.

It is as brutal as also gradually plucking off the two eyes of the potential recruits.

All these are to test for the loyalty of the potential recruits to the military they belong to.

Opposition militaries usually capture opponents and ask them questions about the secrets, the tactics and strategies of the military they belong to.

The brutality through which Pregnickle puts its potential recruits, to test for their loyalty, is the same as those/simulates those inflicted on soldiers from whom opposition armies demand revelation of secrets.

One of the other training underwent by the military students of Pregnickle is that in which a particular thing such as a gun, a rifle or a grenade is kept somewhere in the thick forest.

The military student is asked to look for this thing without a compass.

He also carries about 70 pounds of luggage; he's given a time limit during which the "lost item" must be found.

At the same time, a military troop simulating the opposition army is on their way to capture him alive!

He's subsequently punished brutally for not finding the item!

These training sessions were that brutal!

As brutal as the trainings of the military of Pregnickle were, they can never be compared with notable special forces in the world like:

DELTA FORCE (1ST SFOD-D) – USA

NAVY SEALS – THE UNITED STATES

ALPHA GROUP – RUSSIA

SAYERET MATKAL – ISRAEL

POLISH GROM, POLAND

SPECIAL AIR SERVICE (SAS) – UNITED KINGDOM

NATIONAL GENDARMERIE INTERVENTION GROUP, FRANCE

JOINT TASK FORCE 2 – CANADA

SNOW LEOPARD COMMANDO UNIT, CHINA

SPECIAL NAVAL WARFARE FORCE, SPAIN

EKO COBRA, AUSTRIA

GRUPPO DI INTERVENTO SPECIAL (GIS), ITALY

MARCOS, INDIA

GARUDS (INDIA)

PARA SPECIAL FORCES (PARA SF) INDIA

The whole military investments of Pregnickle, put together, could not in any way overpower or defeat any of the above 15 military squads!

This is alarming and sounds unbelievable!

In one of the attacks whose documentary will be highlighted in a few paragraphs away, some of the armoured tanks got permanently locked by the invading army and the soldiers of Pregnickle got captured in the tanks and got blasted(splenic sequestration crisis).

In the same attack, some of the soldiers died by suffocation in the tanks (splenic sequestration crisis).

Because of an error in target in this same attack, some of the empty tanks were also bomb blasted by the troops of Pregnickle(auto splenectomy).

In some of Pregnickle's war strategies, they sent spies and the Military Intelligence Corps who utilised the LOCKHEED MARTIN RQ-170 SENTINEL and BOEING MQ-25 STINGRAY DRONES, just like Moses sent 12 spies, that included Joshua and Caleb.

[These are synonymous with Memory B Cells, that are involved in surveillance and subsequent mastery of the fight against pathogens by the production of specific antibodies against pathogens to which they have been previously exposed].

The information gathered by these spies and the Military Intelligence Corps were used to defeat the invaders in question.

Sometimes, they deliberately allow war and temporary defeat, so that they can master how their invaders fight and attack(vaccination).

This strategy helped them to win the said countries in subsequent attacks and other invaders who used the same or similar battle strategies.

The beginning of another series of persistent invasions and attacks Pregnickle experienced started in 1880 when news reached opposition armies about a particular bill that was passed.

This bill was passed by the legislative arm of the government of Pregnickle and stated that there should be more children in the military so that there can be more soldiers, naval troops, marines, coast guards, and members of the air force and the space force.

The bill also stipulated that schools offering professional courses and highly technical and cerebral courses reduce the threshold for admitting indigenous students; but raise the bar against foreign students.

In fact the bill particularly stated that all foreign students admitted should be admitted in deceit.

It was in the plan of the school authorities to collect the tuition fee of these students and make sure they do not progress in their studies let alone smell their passing out(official graduation ceremony).

The same bill to lower the threshold for indigenous students and raise the bar against foreign students was passed for all other schools that offered nonprofessional courses.

The bill also stated that the learning conditions and environment for indigenous students be made optimal and to the highest standard possible; so that the students who graduate from the schools can be world class.

Unfortunately this was not the same for foreign students.

The logic behind these bills was that Pregnickle wants to attack neighbouring countries, wipe their race out of the planet earth/ enslave them; and become the most powerful country in the world, having authority and rule over other countries(overpower them both in combat and intellectually).

The legislative arm of the government of Pregnickle meant well by this bill, in that, there was a history of events which happened 1,000 years before that moment: neighbouring countries attacked them ruthlessly in an attempt to wipe them out.

Other countries that were advanced in science and technology also cheated them and carted away mineral resources worth billions of dollars.

Other countries also enslaved them.

The very few of the indigenous people of Pregnickle who escaped the attacks, slavery and intellectual manipulation, procreated and grew into a bigger country between 880AD and 1880.

They have learnt from history and they were not only ready to be defensive; they were more than ready to be offensive.

(The spies who leaked the secret of training more children can also be likened to pregnancy hormones that send messages of, "a baby is coming", throughout the body; the presence of these hormones distort the normal physiology of the pregnant sickle cell patient, just like the information carried by the spies triggered war against Pregnickle).

To consolidate the plans of the legislature of Pregnickle, they consulted the ancient deities of the country(through the chief priests) about which country they could merge with to form an empire.

There were several rituals that were performed, which all started three months before the civilian and military students started academic and training sessions and semesters (trial and error in relationships; three months grace before pregnancy[to stop certain medications and start folic acid]; courting; dating; engagement; relationship; preconceptual care, counselling, medical investigations, family planning etc).

After the three months elapsed, the bill was made a law and was implemented(students started school).

Information reaching the chief priests from the gods(deities) after the rituals was shocking: the only country that qualified to form an empire with Pregnickle was AmunistatA(High Performance Liquid Chromatography[genotype compatibility] stated that the couple are compatible).

AmunistatA had been a very good and close ally of Pregnickle for the past 1000 years.

This country experienced the same attacks, enslavement and intellectual manipulations which Pregnickle experienced.

AmunistatA didn't specialise in training students, having schools, nor teachers; not even children who can be trained to succeed the ancestors.

The habitants, however, were renowned worldwide for being the most advanced country in the fabrication of ammunition used both by the soldiers, the navy, the marines, the coast guards, the air force and the space force.

They fabricate and develop both mechanical weapons, chemical weapons, biological weapons and nuclear weapons[spermatozoa].

All the sea and ocean vessels, aircrafts, armoured vehicles, drones, and ammunition listed and named above, which were in the possession of Pregnickle were all fabricated, designed and developed by AmunistatA!

These bills passed into law already took effect before AmunistatA took steps to design any of those weapons and vehicles.

And the training earlier mentioned in this book including those of the hell week and trust shots, came after the bills were made into law!

The most intelligent authors of textbooks and formal education training materials[spermatozoa] were found only in AmunistatA.

They specialised in producing technologically advanced stationeries[spermatozoa] and classroom learning materials[spermatozoa].

Also, the best military training materials[spermatozoa] were developed in AmunistatA, like you have learnt in the story so far.

So, these bills were made into law; including the proposal of amalgamating[wedding ceremony] the two countries to become an empire[married couple].

The best foods and drinks that facilitate both physical and intellectual prowess were reserved for both the military and the civilian students.

The new law also stipulated that the parents of any students be not allowed to bring food, drinks, consumables, provisions, money or anything at all directly to their children.

The only people permitted by law to do these were the caregivers(placenta) that the teachers (womb) assign to each student(embryo).

The only day when the parents will be able to even see their children is the graduation day(labour and delivery day), the day a caregiver gives up on the assigned student(placenta abruption), the day the student dies(spontaneous abortion),

the day a parent secretly sends drugs prohibited by the chief priests through the caregivers(drugs which cause miscarriages) , the day a student is withdrawn, rusticated, expelled or drops out

(termination of pregnancy because of findings from Preimplantation Genetic Diagnosis, Coelocentesis, Cordocentesis, Amniocentesis etc), the day the chief priests

[medical doctors] discover through the gods [medical investigations] that a student will be a liability or a terror to the empire (birth defects detected through investigations),

or the day a student fails major exams, or the brutal training earlier described (PGD, Coelocentesis, Amniocentesis etc).

Like I said, AmunistatA didn't have schools, classrooms, teachers, lecturers nor military tutors; not even a single child to train or to sponsor in school[no womb, no ovum, no placenta; just spermatozoa].

The deities had orchestrated it before time began, that the manner in which AmunistatA[husband] will have new graduates[babies], new military personnels and new intellectuals[babies] that will succeed its ancestors is to be betrothed[married] to Pregnickle[wife];

and to make sure that the students of Pregnickle get the best of ammunition, textbooks and training materials.

So, in the bill made into law, the children/students of Pregnickle will now bear the identities of both Pregnickle and AmunistatA, because of the tremendous contribution of ammunition, textbooks and training materials from the latter.

SO HOW DID THE OPPOSITION MILITARIES AND COUNTRIES GET TO KNOW ABOUT THE NEW BILL THAT WAS MADE INTO THE LAW?

Unfortunately, some of the military personnels in Pregnickle, acted as spies who worked for some of the opposition militaries.

Some members of the legislature of Pregnickle were also traitors who leaked the masterplan to neighbouring countries.

Before the opposition forces struck, the empire was formed already, bill passed into law and academic and training semesters had already begun.

Also, before the opposition forces struck the empire, the chief priests received information from the deities and instructed accordingly: that there be trees planted around the food processing, food milling, food storage and food preservation factory[liver]; and that very deep drainages be built around the Pentagon: the military headquarters [spleen][to prevent splenic and hepatic sequestration crises].

He added that the Marines, the Navy and the Coast Guards of the opposition forces plan to explode the water reservoirs, and use some magical powers to force water from every nook and cranny of the empire into the food factory and the Pentagon.

As the priests mentioned, this will cause a massive flooding[splenic and hepatic sequestration crises], in the forthcoming attacks.

He also mentioned that if they succeed in doing this, then the empire will lose the energy to exist: its destruction become more imminent[anaemic organ failure secondary to splenic and hepatic sequestration crises] and the survival of fresh graduates beyond day one becomes almost impossible(Liver and spleen span to check for hepatic and splenic sequestration crisis during labour; these crises also occur antenatally, intrapartum and postpartum[especially the peuperum]).

THE BATTLE:

On the first day of school resumption week, deafening sounds were heard as though giant milling machines were on.

These sounds were from the fighter jets, drones, fighter aircrafts, attack aircrafts, trainers, special mission aircrafts, tanker fleet, attack helicopters, and transport aircrafts of the opposition Air Force

[pneumonia, acute chest syndrome, pulmonary hypertension, and pulmonary embolism during pregnancy.

The Air Force represents the immunity of the lungs and everything that enhances the optimal state of the lungs.

The opposition Airforce targets disruption of "airflow" through the four lung pathologies listed above.

It is good to note here that the ammunitions used by the airforce and space force represents the immunity in the pregnant woman to fight against anything that hampers airflow;

ammunitions used by the navy, coast guards and submarines represent the immunity in the pregnant woman to fight against any illness that has to do with body fluids and where body fluids passes through (sepsis, urinary tract infection etc);

ammunitions used by the land forces represents the immunity in the pregnant woman to fight against infections and illnesses of hard tissues and surfaces such as the skin and the mucosa;

The brain is an organ with electrical activities like the transformer and the hydroelectric power plant.

The liver converts glucose to glycogen and helps to store excess food, therefore it represents the food factory.

The spleen is a major organ in the body's defence system; therefore represents the Pentagon, the headquarters of the United States military.

The eyes, the keratinocytes, langerhans cells in the epidermis, dermal mast cells, dendritic cells, T cells, and macrophages, represent the drones and other aircrafts used in the surveillance and reconnaissance missions].

The students heard these deafening sounds and thought that was the norm of day 1 in school.

****

In an attempt to replace the traitor military officers and prominent army personnels who were lost in previous battles, the military absorbed non-natives who were also allies with the two countries(transplant and blood transfusion).

Some of the new non-native military personnels which were absorbed didn't survive because of racism attacks which eliminated them.(graft vs host disease, organ transplant rejection and alloimmunisation after blood transfusion).

At some point the racism attacks even boomeranged against a few indigenous students(Rhesus antibodies in mother's blood against a rhesus positive second baby or first baby in the case of grandmother theory).

Also, the amalgamation of Pregnickle and AmunistatA caused the death of some students of the first and subsequent sets (grandmother theory of the Rhesus antibody; and Rhesus incompatibility of the father and mother respectively) because there were some instructions given by the deity through the chief priest; which the legislative arm missed.

****

BACK TO THE BATTLEFIELD: Surveillance planes (reconnaissance aircrafts or spy planes) of the opposition

Airforce just took off ; and where they hovered, were completely out of sight of the Air Force and space force of Pregnickle.

These planes had surveillance systems that were extremely more sophisticated than Pregnickle's

LOCKHEED MARTIN RQ-170 SENTINEL and BOEING MQ-25 STINGRAY DRONES!

That's really serious, you say?

Unknown to other military members of Pregnickle, the opposition military troops had paid a huge sum to another set of traitors within Pregnickle's troop.

These traitors were supposed to secure the wild animals trained for war.

On the other hand, just before the war began, these traitors[AUTO-] went to the place where the trained lions, tigers, hyenas, foxes and wolves were kept and all trained animals were killed by bleeding them to death[-SPLENECTOMY]: what they were paid to do.[autosplenectomy, caused by repeated deprivation of blood supply to the spleen in vasoocclusive crisis].

There were igneous rock caves that were meant to serve as protection and hiding places where the land troops (army) of Pregnickle lay in ambush for the enemies.

Some of these rock caves also were designed as traps for the invaders.

During this particular war, these igneous rock caves and the strategies designed around them for conquest didn't work out, because the reconnaissance planes already captured the location and the strategies.

Contrary to plans and strategies, some of the soldiers of Pregnickle were trapped by the artificial reactivation of the dormant volcanoes of these igneous rocks by the opposition military's bomb blasts;

These volcanic eruptions trapped the soldiers en masse , locking them permanently in the caves(splenic sequestration crisis); the exact strategy of Pregnickle against the opposition troops (they were caught in the same trap they set).

All efforts to exit the caves and crevices proved abortive and they died from hypoxia and the tremendous heat the volcanoes emitted (they suffocated: splenic sequestration crisis: the red blood cells were destroyed).

The reactivation of the dormant volcanoes was made possible by the firing of missiles very similar to Pregnickle's PRECISION GUIDED MUNITIONS and the MOVING TARGET ARTILLERY ROUNDS!

These missiles were shot by the drones in the earlier mentioned surveillance fleet hovering unknown to anyone in Pregnickle.

The F16 Fighter Jets of the opposition air force were also in their camps set for flight.

The pipes from which Pregnickle's soldiers get their drinkable water were obstructed by the oil deposited by the invaders in the reservoir tanks; these oil deposits coagulated (became solid) and blocked water flow(deep venous thrombosis) both to the soldiers and the plantation from which they fed.

The strategy and plan of the opposition troops was that some of the grease(solidified oils) get dislodged within the pipes and travel long distances(thromboembolism) to obstruct water supplies to the major plantations from where the troops fed; to obstruct water supplies to the air purification plants and the air pumps(lungs; pulmonary embolism), the hydroelectric power plant(brain; ischaemic stroke) and the pumping machines that made sure the entire country (Pregnickle) gets water supply(the heart; a heart attack).

The sewage(liquid waste disposal) system[the kidneys] also had an obstruction of water supply because of the grease dislodgement!

[This caused acute kidney injury!]

The food processing, milling, preservation and storage press(liver), was however not affected by this strategy.

Students continued training sessions as the war proceeded.

There's a temporary shield that the gods have used to protect all military training centres and schools.

This explains why training, academic and school sessions still proceeded despite the ongoing battle.

Their parents, some of whom were civilians, were praying tirelessly for the protection of their children and for the cessation of the attacks.

****

The students are nearing the end of their training term.

Many of them have dropped out because of hell week, trust shots, white noise experience, and pressure and torture to leak the secrets of the military they belonged.

Many dropped out during earlier stages of the training.

Just very few were left, and this secret about how few they have now become was leaked again to the opposition military!

The fact that they'd be passing out in a couple of days was also disclosed to the opposition troops [this leaked secrets represents the signals sent throughout the body by physiological changes at the onset of and during labour; these signals provokes many complications related to either sickle cell, pregnancy or both, just like the leaked secrets provokes further strikes against Pregnickle].

Several months passed, and the war continued with several bomb blasts and bullet injuries.

Several entities were rendered homeless, roofless, destitute, orphans, fatherless and motherless.

Others experienced the deaths of their children.

Several panickings; several places known for hustling and bustling of business activities and road traffic jams were laid in ruins.

Every thinkable place of social gatherings were blasted with Precision Guided Munitions [bombs], except the schools and the military training centres [the womb and some of the children therein were preserved].

There were unavoidable shutdowns of several business centres.

The whole country would have been as silent as a graveyard because of the ruins and the fear of going out of the house;

but for the sounds of bullets, bomb blasts, groanings in the battlefields, activities in the schools and the sounds of helicopters, bush planes, fighter jets, Harrier jump jets, drones, rockets and other space/air crafts.

It's now 9 MONTHS[THE BABY HAS REACHED FULL TERM] since the beginning of the war.

THE LABOUR(CHILDBIRTH)

The air force and the space force of the invading military made sure that the speed of the wind be rapid and irregular[tachypnoea and dyspnoea respectively during labour] ; and that the intensity of sunshine be significantly increased[fever during labour].

They succeeded in doing the former by firing bullets at the colossal air pumps[lungs] installed at the lowest part of Pregnickle's atmosphere (the troposphere).

The air pumps were supposed to ensure that the inhabitants of Pregnickle+AmunistatA had access to abundant oxygen and therefore prevent the crumbling of the empire.

The irregular speed of the wind caused by the enemies, like the Chief priests professed, was already causing the empire to crumble.

"This will also determine if the new graduates[foetuses at childbirth] of the empire will survive or not", a Chief priest mentioned.

"It only takes an immediate replacement of these air pumps(ventilators) to prevent the empire from being a forgotten hero ", another Chief priest added.

The enemies attempted to also blast the electric transformers[brain] which supplied electric power to these air pumps; but the space force's and the air force's aircrafts were actually around these space transformers and they were all set to blast any invaders who came close.

The empire's air and space force were proactive because of the words of one of the chief priests: "if the invading troops succeed in blasting the space transformers, then the empire comes to an end immediately!"[brain death secondary to stroke].

"Not even another transformer nor air pumps would be able to save the day!", the priests added.

So, all the troops that were on their way to blast the transformers[brain death], were roasted in the blast from Pregnickle's PRECISION GUIDED MUNITIONS; they didn't succeed!

Both in the space (respiratory rate) and within the empire (pulse oximetry), there were anemometers(respiratory rate) installed in order to know the speed of wind entering from the space and another instrument(pulse oximeter) also made sure that the oxygen concentration was high enough for optimal access to the inhabitants of the empire.

In some of the schools and the classrooms[wombs] where the new graduates were produced(on the graduation day), the opposition space force also caused tremendous snowing [hypothermia in the mother and the baby] which was unprecedented in the country.

The Navy, the Marines and the Coast Guard made sure that on the same day of graduation, water from the reservoir ceased to be supplied for drinking[dehydration]; and that each school, classroom and teachers that orchestrated the

qualification of the graduates be either bled to death[postpartum haemorrhage]
or suffocated with a flood[fluid overload].

Because of the rate at which water wasted in this particular flood, the machines that were responsible for pumping the water[the heart] became overworked making them to either have a faster rate[tachycardia from hypovolemia], slower rate[bradycardia from hypovolemia] or irregular rate of pumping[arrythmias from hypovolemia].

As a matter of fact some of these machines "kicked the bucket"[heart failure] that same day.

In some parts of Pregnickle, the Navy, the Marines and the Coast guards of the opposition forces, on this graduation[childbirth] day also drastically reduced the rate of water supply to both the parents, the teachers and the caregivers [dehydration during labour].

Just a day before the passing out of the successful military students, all the prominent soldiers and heads of the military (the Commander-in-Chief of all the Armed Forces, The Secretary Of Defense, Deputy Secretary of Defense, The Chairman of the Joint Chiefs of Staff, The Vice Chairman of the Joint Chiefs of Staff,
Generals of the Army, Generals, the Lieutenant Generals, the Major Generals, the Brigadier Generals, the Colonels, the Lieutenant Colonels, the Majors and the Captains; the

Generals of the Air force; the Fleet Admiral of the Navy and the Coast Guard; the General of the Marine Corps Master Chief Petty Officers of the Navy) were killed by sleet or ice pellets(rain that got solidified [blood coagulation or clot formation: thrombosis] before reaching the earth). [Ischaemic stroke from a thromboembolic event; this didn't cause brain death]

They died, not because they weren't physically strong enough to withstand common sleets /ice pellets; but because the space force already knew the abominations that the gods said these top officials should avoid: sleets/ ice pellets during a war.

So, the space force of the opposition military knew about this and used it against them by causing tremendous lowering of the temperature in space and the precipitation of a downpour on the troops including the top officials.

Mr. President, the Commander-in-Chief of all the Armed Forces, died because of this abomination too!

NOT ALL STUDENTS MADE IT TO THE NINTH MONTH

When news got to the civilian and military schools about the death of the top officials of the armed forces and other things that transpired in the battlefield, some of the students who were being trained (military school) began to lose focus and concentration in their training.

The aforementioned favourable learning and training conditions in the schools and classrooms didn't matter anymore because of the ruins, the war and the fear in the students.

For this reason and/or other reasons, some of them:

....

1. could no longer advance in their military career(foetal growth restriction);

2. Some of their caregivers went to join the others in the battle field[placenta abruption].

3. were sent prematurely/preterm to
the battlefield. [Preterm/premature delivery].

4. some were overfed from the food their parents couldn't eat, trained extra hard and were recommended by the authority for double promotion (high birth weight, secondary to gestational diabetes);

5. had earlier graduation (delivery earlier than EDD[expected day of delivery] because of foetal growth restriction and high birth weight).

6. had sponsorship of tuition and graduation fee(an assisted delivery: Caesarean section).

7. passed on trial because they were overqualified and acquired too many skills within too short a time(gestational diabetes which caused high birth weight in the babies).

8. Some had an opposite experience: they struggled to catch up with other students, but they didn't need any sponsorship for their tuition or graduation fee.[low birth weight].

9. Some of them couldn't cope anymore and they died during rigorous training sessions. [Miscarriage].

10. Some were withdrawn from the school because they lost the financial support of their parents, sponsors for tuition fees or/and caregivers assigned to them by their instructors decided to give up on them (Placenta Abruption).

7. Some of them sustained permanent injuries/ traumas that rendered them disabled (either physical or mental health disability in newborns: birth defects).

8. Some of their parents missed important instructions about drugs/medications to give and those not to be given. This caused some of them to die or have physical or mental health disability.(Angiotensin Receptor Blockers,

Angiotensin Converting Enzyme, hydroxyurea, folic acid deficiency and their sequelae; Neural Tube Defects).

9. Some died from the chemical weapons that the opposition Airforce sprayed into the air.

[birth asphyxia, foetal distress, HIE(hypoxic ischemic encephalopathy){the brains of some students got damaged by the unavailability of enough oxygen from the air pump},

Respiratory distress syndrome (some graduated prematurely and could not breathe well because of what the chief priests have predicted about the students who do not complete the stipulated training period)].

10. Some who were ripe for graduation would have had to stay for extra weeks, because the parents couldn't pay for their graduation fee.(the mother couldn't push).

Some of the wealthy parents were able to save the day and pay for their graduation and induction.(Caesarean section).

11. Some were partly assisted by other students' parents by paying part of their induction and graduation fee (prostaglandin, balloon catheters, artificially breaking the waters & oxytocin[induction of labour]).

12. Others had this partial assistance even before they were ripe for graduation (37-38 weeks), because they and their

parents couldn't forge further than this period.[earlier delivery].

The authority was liberal enough to give them that opportunity.

These students were grateful because some parents couldn't even afford the cost of enrolling their children into a formal education setting (infertility; which is very common among female sickle cell warriors).

13. Some of the caregivers assigned to these students, for reasons which couldn't be controlled, served as deterrents to the graduation of the students they cared for (Placenta Previa, an obstruction of the uterine cervix by the placenta).

****

In one of the consultations made with the Chief priests long before now, a tragic information was reiterated!

Pregnickle, from the beginning of time had experienced scale deposits(precipitates and crystals formed from the calcium and magnesium salts in hard water) [sickle-shaped red blood cells] which occlude tiny pipes and terminal pipes that supplied water to both animals, plants and humans.[vasoocclusive events in sickle cell].

A quick note before we continue: the colour of the water that rains from the skies, flows in the streams, wells, rivers, lakes and other water bodies in Pregnickle is colour wine; it looks like blood[this typifies the blood in the body of the sickle cell pregnant woman].

The colour of the water however does not affect the lives of humans, plants and animals in an adverse manner.

Some of the plantations that needed irrigation from this water source have withered because of this deprivation of water.(precipitates obstructed the pipes: sickle cell Vaso occlusive events].

Back to the tragic information reiterated by the Chief Priests[doctors]; before time began they had asserted and now repeat the assertion, that the precipitates formed in this water will block the water flow to the new schools, and will affect the productivity of the teachers[the womb],

the caregivers[placenta] and by extension the quality of the students and the education/training they receive.

(blood flow to the foetus through the placenta is obstructed because of the sickle cells; fertility is hampered for the same reason evident by lower ovarian reserve; several complications earlier highlighted as seen in the foetus).

"As a matter of fact, because of the blockage of water supply, the time span or length of time during which these schools' accreditation will last for will be reduced;

after some time, the schools will not be recognised anymore as settings capable of delivering formal education or training to students", the priests added.[early menopause].

The students were supposed to spend 40 weeks($\approx$9 months) in their training. But they were meant to take exams:

before gaining admission into the school (Entrance Examination) [Preimplantation Genetic Diagnosis]

at 7th–9th week [Coelocentesis for aspiration of coelomic fluid]

at 10th-12th week [Chorionic Villus Sampling]

at 14th-15th week [Amniocentesis]; and

at 18th-19th week [DNA analysis or foetal blood sampling by cordocentesis]

Some students didn't pass the entrance examination.

Some students got withdrawn/ dropped out from the school at 7th-9th week; 10th-12th week 14th to 15th week; 18th to

19th week; because their conducts suggested that they'll put their parents to shame if they were allowed to graduate.[birth defects and anomalies].

Plus, they didn't pass the exams conducted at weeks 7-9, 10-12, 14-15, and 18-19.

The fate of some were already highlighted in several paragraphs away: they dropped out because of the hell week training, trust shots and torture to reveal their military secrets!

Some of these examinations which they didn't pass were conducted in the course of some of the trainings that led to them being dropped out.

[intrauterine investigations done on the foetus].

There were some antidotes that the gods recommended for cancelling out the effects of the precipitates in the water of Pregnickle.

Some of the Chief priests, however, disobeyed the recommendations of the gods and this caused tremendous sparks in all the transformers supplying electricity in Pregnickle.

[Managing pain (secondary to vasoocclusive events) with pethidine is strongly associated with seizures: abnormal electrical activities in the brain very synonymous with sparks in a transformer].

Some of the recommendations of the gods however also had some minimal risks: the children being trained in the military schools would come down with a temporary heart problem. [Opioids given for pain relief during late pregnancy, causes withdrawal symptoms in the foetus; this is characterised by a temporary reduction in the foetal heart rate].

Just as the gods predicted, Pregnickle experienced similar electric sparks on its transformers because of an increased pressure in the flow of water within Pregnickle's pipes[This illustrates eclampsia, a condition in which there's raised blood pressure and proteinuria during pregnancy which is accompanied by seizure episodes].

Kindly note that the caregivers of each military student represent the placenta, a tissue responsible for supplying nutrients and oxygen to the growing foetus.

Just like the placenta is like a middleman between the mother and the growing foetus; so are the caregivers between the parents and the military students.

The teachers and the schools represent the womb[the environment most conducive for foetal development and growth].

The successful military trainees who qualify for graduation are still awaiting the date on which they'll pass out.

These new military graduates-to-be had to undergo a ritual of taking fruits that are juicy + fresh cow milk for 6 months[exclusive breastfeeding]; then this can later be taken along with other diets for another 1 1/2 years[breastfeeding for another 1½ years + other quality diets].

This ritual also stipulates that the parents of these graduates be responsible for plucking these fruits; also making the fresh cow milk available and feeding their respective children.[mothers must feed their newborns and have a bonding with them from the first hour of birth].

These parents would also be responsible for making sure that organic fertilisers are professionally applied to the plants bearing the fruits; and that the cows that are milked in these rituals be well fed with the very best of diets.[mothers of these new-borns must be equally adequately fed, to enhance quality breast milk production and to optimise the general health of the mother].

****

LABOUR CONTINUES

The day of passing out has been announced.

Another set of opposition military forces have been notified of this graduation date by the traitors.

[The leak of this information is synonymous with the signals the body sends to the nook and crannies of the pregnant woman's body. The signal gives a response of warfare: splenic and hepatic sequestration crises, acute chest syndrome, pulmonary embolism, pulmonary hypertension, ischaemic stroke, deep venous thrombosis, dysfunctional respiratory rate & pulse rate, glucosuria & proteinuria on urinalysis, increased blood pressure, haemorrhage, preeclampsia, eclampsia, gestational diabetes, pneumonia, urinary tract infection, acute kidney injury, and every single complications that are seen in the pregnant sickle cell patient. It's a complex physiology of events that bring about these pathologies].

This new set of opposition troops represent the second batch of troops that'd be invading Pregnickle in the last nine months.

These troops were from another country entirely.

They were the ALPHA GROUP (RUSSIA)!

They had almost the same kind of targets and strategies with the previous opposition troops.

They were able to break through the empire and their first target which they headed for was the hydroelectric power plant of the country(this supplies power to the empire through the electric transformers in each community).[The brain and the nervous system]

The power plant was responsible for powering the water plants(pumping machines: the heart); and by extension the main food processing and preservation plants, the water purification plants, and the sewage system.[the liver and the kidneys respectively].

The Alpha Group damaged the hydroelectric power plant and some of the transformers (another stroke); with the same mechanism, they destroyed the locomotive aspects of the water plants (pumping machine).(Myocardial Infarction/heart attack which almost lead to a Cardiac Arrest).

They effected these damages by the grease mechanism[thromboembolic events] and by influencing the blockage of the penstock(a pipe) of the hydroelectric water plant . This stopped the flow of the water and therefore ceased the turbine from producing electricity.[ischaemic stroke]

They also influenced how the fuel pumps were clogged(venous thromboembolic events); this caused the shut down of more electrical systems (stroke; more infarcts in the brain from thromboembolism) and more sections of the water plant (pumping machines)[Myocardial Infarction and Cardiac Arrest].

Another set of opposition troops that were against Pregnickle, named, the DELTA FORCE (1ST SFOD-D) & the NAVY SEALS of THE UNITED STATES,

succeeded in blocking the fuel filter of the mechanical system powering the water plant (acute kidney injury).

They represent the third and fourth batches of the opposition troops respectively!

In the hydroelectric power stations, the Oxygen Injection Processes which inject oxygen into the air intake of the engines were also clogged by the Delta force and the Navy SEALS of the United States!

The air force of the first opposition military troops in the F16 fighter jets earlier mentioned have taken off already for attack after 9 solid months!

These aircrafts didn't attack with the conventional mechanical weapons this time!

They went chemical by spraying chlorine, phosgene, and mustard gases into the air and this killed the civilian parents enmasse.[they weakened the immunity of their respiratory system-pneumonia and Acute Chest Syndrome].

Pregnickle couldn't dominate the airspace of the battlefield during this phase of the war!

All its aircrafts including the almighty reconnaissance LOCKHEED MARTIN RQ-170 SENTINEL and BOEING MQ-25 STINGRAY; and the weaponised drones were brought to nought by a MOVING TARGET ARTILLERY ROUND of the United States Navy SEALS and the Delta force!

It wasn't that easy bringing these powerful aircrafts down, but the opposition did[sickle cell proliferative retinopathy; surveillance systems of the body's immune system were brought down: immunosuppression. Aircraft defence also represents the defence of the lung's immunity system. Pneumonia invariably has set in].

Pregnickle wasn't prepared at all for a chemical weapon attack or defence.

All the strange strategies deployed by the opposition militaries, Pregnickle wasn't familiar with nor prepared for any!

****

Despite the fact that the legislative arm of Pregnickle desired more students in the military, there was a clause that the Chief priests added:

"The number of students that can be admitted in a lifetime by each military school is 1,000,000; which makes the slots for trainable students very limited. We recommend this because if we keep enrolling students into the schools, there'd be triggers of war from the opposition army. Any of these wars could mark the end of Pregnickle".

(These limited slots for trainable students in Pregnickle are synonymous with measures taken in Family Planning.

Family planning for the sickle cell woman cannot be overemphasised because it keeps her away from all the brutal complications encountered during pregnancy).

****

Some water pipes were blasted and shattered (nausea and vomiting) by IBMs, PGMs and MTARs shot from one of the vessels in the ocean.

Because of this, the community lost a lot of water which affected the health of the parents[dehydration during labour](like what happened in the parable of the foolish farmer in Northern Nigeria) as there was no water to drink (mother).

As the water gushed out from the broken pipes, some parents attempted to drink excessively so that it can take them for the next few days; all unfortunately died from a heart failure/pulmonary edema/pulmonary hypertension, secondary to fluid overload.

The central tanks that supplied hot water to the communities in this country were also damaged[hypothermia].

Some military personnels of Pregnickle were trapped in live wire traps set by the third and fourth batch invaders.

The filters that purify the drinking water in the Southern parts of Pregnickle, were made porous by the same troops and this allowed poisonous particles[proteins in the urine] into the drinkable water(pre-eclampsia).

The invaders were able to do this by narrowing, twisting and bending the pipes that supplied water to all students in Pregnickle[remodelling of the blood vessels in the placenta; a mechanism established as the cause of preeclampsia]; thereby increasing the pressure of water flow through the filter.

Because of this pressure increase, the pipes very close to the transformers got broken and there was a tremendous flooding that covered these transformers in Pregnickle.

This affected the supply of electricity to many parts of the country! (haemorrhagic stroke).

As the war proceeded, and despite the fact that some military heroes of Pregnickle had fallen, they didn't retreat or give way to the opposition troops.

As a matter of fact, they even assured the Commander-in-Chief of all the Armed Forces(Mr. President) before his death, that the war is under control and that the security of the students [who would be graduating in a couple of hours] [term babies] is guaranteed!

"There's absolutely no need to stop the passing out parade of the successful candidates", they added.

Some of the troops of Pregnickle who didn't get the information about the poisoned drinkable water, drank this water.

What this poison did was that it made the soldiers lose appetite and they starved to death despite the availability of food in abundance.

[inability of the cells to make use of glucose in gestational diabetes. In gestational diabetes, insulin is available but unfortunately cannot be used to drive in glucose seamlessly into the cells of the pregnant sickle cell patient.

Ewedu is a kind of soup that has a lubricating effect in the throat, while swallowing some foods[e.g Amala] in West Africa! Like Ewedu is to Amala, so is insulin to glucose: "a lubricant".

But in situations where Ewedu is overcooked, it loses its lubricating quality. This is what happens in gestational diabetes; the insulin can no longer drive glucose into the cells. Insulin " loses its lubricating quality", hence the term insulin resistance].

Because the military troops who were poisoned could no longer feed, the plantation they should have fed from was wasted(excessive glucose in the blood which became useless and wasted because of insulin resistance in gestational diabetes).

The wasted plantation[excessive blood glucose] was disposed of eventually through the waste management authority(glucosuria: this is also known as presence of glucose in the urine. It's a feature in gestational diabetes. The body had to get rid of the excessive glucose in the blood through urine).

****

The increased pressure of water flow in some of the pipes was alarmingly high, that this pressure broke some pipes and caused a flood which damaged more parts of the hydroelectric power plant(haemorrhagic stroke).

Some military troops in some of Pregnickle's camps drowned and suffocated(haemorrhagic stroke) because of this flood; in some camps, this flood caused the plantation from which the respective troops fed to stop growing(haemorrhagic stroke).

But for the proactiveness of the heads of the Navy, the Marines, the Coast Guards, the army, the air force and the space force, the information about the new bill that was made a law in Pregnickle; which the spies leaked would have marked the end of Pregnickle!

The winning was by a whisker however, with a lot of graduates(babies), many parents, tutors, trainers and instructors lost to the battles!

Pregnickle managed to produce 100 world class, physically and mentally resilient and brutal military graduates!

These could withstand and resist all the world's top 15 military squads, put together!

Pregnickle and AmunistatA lived happily ever after as married couples/an empire, with several other batches of armed forces successfully graduating and surviving the brutality that defines their training!

THE END.

WATCH OUT FOR PART 2 OF BATTLE IN MY WOMB TO GET BETTER EXPLANATION FOR THE MEDICAL TERMINOLOGIES IN THIS BOOK AND THE FUTURE OF PREGNICKLE'S MILITARY WITH ITS ENEMIES!

THE MEDICAL TERMINOLOGIES AND HOW EACH RELATES TO THE PARABLES, SIMILES, METAPHORS AND OTHER FIGURES OF SPEECH USED WILL BE CLEARLY EXPLAINED IN THE PART 2 OF THIS BOOK.

IN THIS PART 2, YOU'LL GET TO KNOW HOW I CAME ABOUT THE FICTIONAL NAMES, PREGNICKLE AND AMUNISTATA TOO….. !

CHAPTER 3

ACADEMIC ASPECT OF THIS BOOK

The sickle cell girl child

The sickle cell girl child is prone to infertility because of multiple infarctions in her ovaries.

There's incidence of increased pain during menstruation, heavy flow of blood per menstrual cycle and delayed puberty.

PS: Gynaecologists still don't believe there's a relationship between menstruation, menstrual pain and sickle cell Vaso occlusive bone pain crisis.

They have not been able to see the relationship between menstruation, menstrual pain and crisis.

And the reason is they cannot explain the pathophysiology just yet.

I asked one of them here in Nigeria, he said there's no relationship.

But because of 3 other SCD patients' reports and other documented cases, I documented it in my second book on SCD and this book also.

The pathophysiology for menstrual pain; I was told, is not the same as the pathophysiology of sickle cell pain.

Also, it's common for male doctors not to believe that there is a relationship between menstrual pain and sickle cell crisis.

Menstrual pain triggers the crisis.

THE MANAGEMENT OF MENSTRUAL PAIN THAT COMES WITH MENSTRUAL FLOW AND WHICH TRIGGERS SC CRISIS.

If the menstrual pain is severe and persistent, hormonal birth control to halt period is a good option.

THE PRECONCEPTUAL CARE

Partner haemoglobin genotype testing using high performance liquid chromatography or point of care test.

Commencement of Folic Acid 5mg daily, 3 months before pregnancy (this is a routine which must have been long commenced for a SCD patient anyway).

Discontinuation of hydroxyurea(3 months before pregnancy), angiotensin receptor blockers, angiotensin converting enzyme inhibitors(two classes of antihypertensives used sometimes to prevent hypertension complicated by proteinuria in sickle cell disease) and other medications contraindicated in pregnancy.

During each adult haematology clinic visits, adequate information (about how sickle cell disease affect the pregnancy status and vice versa)must be given to all adolescent girl who have confirmed their intention to conceive.

Contraception options should be clearly spelt out to patient during these routine haematology clinic appointments so that patient can be persuaded to explore their preference. Contraception at this stage of adolescence prevents patients from carrying babies that might be having sickle cell disease, thalassemias or any other genetic anomaly.

Patients must be screened for end organic damage such as stroke, sickle cell retinopathy (proliferative retinopathy), sickle cell nephropathy and sickle cell hepatopathy.

They should be screened for pulmonary hypertension too with echocardiography.

Screening for iron overload and aggressive chelation(mopping up of iron load) should be instituted if there's significant iron overload.

The option of surrogacy, in vitro fertilisation and ECTOLIFE®(the newest and the most advanced technology in the world[artificial womb] for nurturing a foetus from fertilisation through embryonic stage till term) should be given to the couple. The first and third options avail the sickle cell woman the opportunity of having a child without being subjected to the multitude of complications.

Invitro fertilisation avails the patient the opportunity to have Preimplantation Genetic Diagnosis. The latter lets the couple know if the oocyte or the embryo have genetic disorders like sickle cell disease.

This makes sure that the most promising sperm fertilises the most promising ovum.

Full blood count is a must, so that the Physicians can know what the baseline figures of the PCV, white blood cells and platelets are; this will guide the managing team on deciding whether patient needs a blood transfusion (in case of PCV reduction below baseline) or needs to be treated for an infection or sepsis (when white blood cells rise above baseline).

Screening for cervical cancer, breast cancer, syphilis, HIV, Hepatitis B surface antigen, Hepatitis C Virus, other sexually transmitted diseases, and other vertically transmitted infections (i.e infections that can be transmitted from mother to child in the womb).

They should be vaccinated against cervical cancer, encapsulated organisms such as Streptococcus pneumoniae, Neisseria meningitidis, Influenza and Hepatitis B. Haemophilus influenzae type B + Conjugated Meningococcal C vaccines should be given as a single dose if they have not received it as part of primary vaccination.

Pneumococcal vaccine should be given every 5 years.

Some of these vaccines prevent recurrent sepsis which is a trigger for a vaso occlusive bone pain crisis.

Influenza and "swine flu" vaccines should be taken annually.

Penicillin prophylaxis or Erythromycin (if patient is allergic to Penicillin) should be given to also prevent recurrent sepsis, a trigger to recurrent vaso occlusive crisis.

ADMINISTRATION AND PRESCRIPTION OF PENICILLIN SHOULD HOWEVER FOLLOW THE UNITED KINGDOM GUIDELINES OUTLINED IN RESPECT TO HYPOSPLENIC SICKLE CELL PATIENTS;

because there's no research yet done on the effectiveness of Penicillin in adult sickle cell patients (as is the case with paediatric sickle cell patients).

The option of Preimplantation Genetic Diagnosis which can be done during invitro fertilisation should be explained clearly to the patient.

This investigation allows the couple to know if there are any anomaly in the embryo or the oocyte. If there are, the embryo will not be implanted.

Red blood cell antibodies in the mother's blood, such as Rhesus, Kell, etc must be ascertained and if necessary, mopped up by a procedure known as Apheresis/Pheresis.

This prevents erythroblastosis fetalis(Haemolytic Disease of the NewBorn); a condition in which the red blood cells of the foetus are attacked by the antibodies in the mother's blood.

Monitoring the foetus with an ultrasound scan can also help in detecting if the foetus is already being affected by the incompatibility between the mother's and baby's blood type.

Early delivery might be planned by the obstetrician depending on the outcome of this ultrasound scan.

ANTENATAL CARE.

Patients should be warned about overexertion, excessive exercise, dehydration and extremes of temperature (too hot or too cold weather conditions). They are triggers of a vaso occlusive bone pain crisis, which patient should avoid.

They should also be informed about the other triggers of a vaso occlusive bone pain crisis: malaria and sepsis. Patients must sleep under insecticide treated net, must be on malaria prophylaxis (200mg proguanil daily) and must have all infection prophylaxis and vaccines listed in preconceptual care taken except live attenuated vaccines which are deferred until after delivery.

If there's laboratory evidence of iron deficiency(very rare in SCD), patient can be commenced on iron supplements like Fersolate®.

Vomiting is top on the list of the causes of dehydration during pregnancy.

Vomiting can be prevented by:

Vitamin B-6 supplements.

Ginger supplements, foods and drinks.

Eating less spicy and greasy foods, eating more complex carbohydrates (bread and pasta).

Eating fruits and leafy green vegetables.

Sipping cool and clear beverages e.g. carbonated drinks.

Taking light snacks immediately after waking up from bed.

Taking meals in smaller bits and very often.

Using acupressure wrist band, and drugs such as doxylamine (Unisom®).

If symptoms continue, patient might require prescription anti-nausea medications like prochlorperazine or chlorpromazine.

Identify the triggers and avoid them or manage them. Some smells, tastes or even noise can trigger a nausea and vomiting. If you unavoidably encounter a trigger, sniff on a slice of lemon or suck on a mint.

If vomiting is still severe and still not resolving, parenteral feeding may be the best bet so that the mother and child can survive.

First two trimesters (first 6 months of pregnancy), patient must present to the antenatal clinic every two weeks where her blood pressure, packed cell volume (PCV) and urinalysis must be done.

The BP and the urinalysis is done to be sure the woman doesn't have preeclampsia.

Preeclampsia is simply high blood pressure associated with pregnancy with simultaneous evidence of protein in the urine (proteinuria).

On a good day, the kidney is a filter that doesn't allow large molecules from the blood to pass through it into urine.

But, in preeclampsia and many kidney pathologies, large molecules like proteins can find their ways through the kidneys.

MIDSTREAM URINE CULTURE should be done every month, because urinary tract infection is the third most common infection experienced by the sickle cell pregnant woman.

Sepsis and pneumonia top the list.

A drop in the PCV may be indicative of a Splenic Sequestration Crisis>Aplastic Crisis>Acute Haemolytic Crisis.

Please kindly see the definition of these crises in my third book: "Sickle Cell Unmasked".

A drop in Haemoglobin Concentration below 9.5g/dL or 3% reduction from previous antenatal values requires an urgent blood transfusion.

It is the duty of the physician seeing the patient to measure the spleen and liver span. If the spleen and the liver are enlarged and there's concurrent drop in PCV, then, this drop is most likely to be caused by a splenic sequestration or hepatic sequestration crisis.

If reticulocyte count is reduced with a concurrent drop in PCV, then it is most likely Aplastic Crisis.

Patient need to be isolated if diagnosed with Aplastic Crisis because it's associated with an infection with Parvovirus B19 virus.

The antenatal sickle crises and complications might follow this order in terms of how common they are: Vaso occlusive bone pain crisis> Acute Chest Syndrome> Pneumonia>Urinary Tract Infection.

In this order in terms of how common they are, we have the following too as life-threatening complications that can be experienced by the sickle cell pregnant woman: pulmonary embolism> stroke>aplastic anaemia>acute haemolytic crisis>splenic sequestration crisis.

The sickle cell pregnant woman should not be managed in a primary nor secondary health care centre except if these centres have haematologists who have special interest in sickle cell disease, obstetricians that have a track record of successfully managing high risk pregnancies, midwives and anaesthetists that are very vast and experienced; and INTENSIVE CARE UNIT FACILITIES.

Bullets 2, 3, 6, 8, 9, 11 in the preconceptual care section, if not already done, can be done/commenced as soon as the patient is seen in the antenatal clinic.

For couples who presented late after conception, and who would want to get rid of a baby with sickle cell disease, or other anomaly, diagnosis of the developing child to check for any birth or genetic anomaly is still possible at:

i. 7th–9th week [Coelocentesis by aspiration of coelomic fluid]

    ii. 10th-12th week [Chorionic Villus Sampling]

    iii. 14th-15th week [Amniocentesis]

    iv. 18th-19th week [DNA analysis or foetal blood sampling by cordocentesis]

For every single visit to the antenatal clinic, the vital signs which include the temperature, blood pressure, respiratory rate, pulse rate, and the oxygen saturation (spO2) must be done!

The temperature helps to pick easily any underlying infections such as Urinary Tract Infection, Pneumonia or Acute Chest Syndrome.

Acute Chest Syndrome and Pneumonia have cough and shortness of breath as additional clinical features.

The spO2 if less than 95 of 100, and if the respiratory rate is high, then a clinical suspicion of Acute Chest Syndrome, Pneumonia or pulmonary embolism must be in place and emergency treatment instituted immediately!

Increased blood pressure is strongly associated with preeclampsia as I have earlier stated.

If blood pressure and proteinuria has concurrent seizure episodes, then eclampsia is diagnosed and must be treated immediately.

Low molecular weight heparin (clot prevention agent) should be given DURING ANY ANTENATAL HOSPITAL ADMISSIONS because both sickle cell disease and the pregnancy state predispose the pregnant woman to clot formation (HYPERCOAGULATION STATE: DEEP VENOUS THROMBOSIS) which can dislodge from the veins and travel into the lungs (PULMONARY EMBOLISM) and thereafter to the brain (ISCHAEMIC STOKE).

The use of GRADUATED COMPRESSION STOCKINGS of appropriate strength is a must in a pregnant sickle cell woman because of the same reason highlighted above.

ULTRASOUND SCANS, DATES AND INDICATIONS:

Viability scan at 7–9 weeks of gestation.

Routine first-trimester scan (11–14 weeks of gestation).

Detailed anomaly scan at 20 weeks of gestation.

Serial foetal biometry scans (growth scans), EVERY WEEK FROM 24 WEEKS OF GESTATION.

At about the 20th week of pregnancy, Intrauterine Foetal Growth Restriction(IUFGR) can be diagnosed using ultrasound scanning.

It's an obstetric complication common in the pregnant sickle cell patient just like the following obstetric complications are:

OBSTETRIC COMPLICATIONS WHOSE INCIDENCE HEIGHTENS IN A PREGNANT SICKLE CELL WOMAN.

Preeclampsia.
Eclampsia.

Gestational Diabetes.
Intrauterine Foetal Growth Restriction.
High Birth Weight.
Low Birth Weight.
Preterm Delivery.
Placenta Abruption.
Placenta Previa.
Perinatal Mortality.

Detailed explanation of these terminologies will be made in the part 2 of this book.

Hypoxic Ischaemic Encephalopathy, Birth Asphyxia and other causes of neonatal morbidity and mortality which are peculiar to children born by sickle cell mothers, will be equally and extensively explained.

Prophylactic blood transfusion, which is a former practice, is no longer indicated, because there's no evidence that this improves maternal or foetal outcomes.

Blood typing ahead of acute anaemia or sickle cell complications is extremely important as well, so that when the need arise, blood or blood products can be available for transfusion immediately.

Low dose aspirin(75mg daily) which reduces the risk of preeclampsia (by reducing the Thromboxane Prostacyclin ratio), should be commenced by the 12th week of pregnancy except the patient has underlying states that makes aspirin contraindicated.

For a sickle cell Vaso occlusive crisis, diclofenac and other Nonsteroidal Anti-inflammatory Drugs should not be take before 12th week nor after 28th week of pregnancy. This class of drugs are safe between 12th- 28th week of pregnancy.

Depending on pain severity and other factors, paracetamol, dihydrocodeine (df118®)co-codamol, or morphine are safe before 12th week and after 28th week of pregnancy. Kindly check the bonus section to have an overview of how pain is generally managed in sickle cell patients with addiction prevention in mind.

If opioids are administered during late pregnancy, the foetal heart rate might be slow and the foetus at birth may show signs of withdrawal symptoms; this is not a thing to worry about because there'll be spontaneous resolution with time.

The risk of losing a patient because of the sedative effects of parenteral opioid administration is high.

During pregnancy, if parenteral(intravenous, intramuscular or subcutaneous) opioids are administered for severe pain;

monitor pain, sedation, vital signs, respiratory rate and oxygen saturation every 20–30 minutes until pain is controlled and signs are stable;

then monitor every 2 hours (hourly if receiving parenteral opiates);

Give a rescue doses of analgesia if required;

If respiratory rate is less than 10/minute, omit maintenance analgesia; consider naloxone;

Consider reducing analgesia after 2–3 days and replacing injections with equivalent dose of oral analgesia.

Because of the side effects of opioids, such as constipation, itching (pruritus), nausea and vomiting; laxatives, antipruritic and antiemetic drugs should be prescribed as needed.

MANAGING OTHER COMPLICATIONS OF SICKLE DURING ANTENATAL CARE

SEPSIS:

Vital signs monitoring

Intravenous Fluoroquinolones(Levofloxacin for example)/ Cephalosporins (ceftriaxone).

IV Paracetamol 600mg stat.

Adequate hydration[Normal Saline 60mls/kg/24hrs or 3L per 24hrs] and oxygen.

Hospital admission.

URINARY TRACT INFECTION

Midstream Urine Microscopy Culture and Sensitivity.

Empirical antibiotics.

Definitive antibiotic therapy after culture and sensitivity results are out.

Vital signs monitoring.

Adequate hydration and oxygen.

ACUTE CHEST SYNDROME AND PNEUMONIA

Pneumonia must be treated simultaneously with acute chest syndrome because both cannot be differentiated clinically.

A chest x-ray with new infiltrates in the lungs is diagnostic of acute chest syndrome.

Patient placed on a monitor for Vital signs.

SPO2 monitoring.

Ventilator support if spO2 is less than 95%.

Respiratory Rate must be monitored too.

If this ranges between 35 & 40 per minute, then the patient must be moved to the intensive care unit.

Haemoglobin Concentration must not be less than 9.5g/dL.

If there is severe anaemia of about 18% PCV, then, there must be RED BLOOD CELL TRANSFUSION till PCV becomes 27-28%.

IN THE EVENT THAT THE HAEMATOLOGY UNIT IS PRESENT, EXCHANGE BLOOD TRANSFUSION IS BETTER FOR BOTH PNEUMONIA AND ACUTE CHEST SYNDROME IF THERE'S SEVERE ANAEMIA [ABOUT 18% PCV].

Monitoring of other vital signs.

Adequate hydration [60mls/kg/24hrs] with a fluid chart to prevent fluid overload.

AZITHROMYCIN AND AUGMENTIN combination are the antibiotics of choice.

If chest infection [pneumonia] or symptoms in Acute Chest Syndrome is very severe, FLUOROQUINOLONES [e.g LEVOFLUOXACIN] are good options.

ACUTE STROKE

Emergency EBT (Exchange Blood Transfusion)

ACUTE SPLENIC/HEPATIC SEQUESTRATION CRISES

Simple Blood Transfusion.

APLASTIC CRISIS

Simple Blood Transfusion.

ACUTE HAEMOLYTIC CRISIS

Treat the cause of the haemolysis(malaria or sepsis).

Simple Blood Transfusion.

VASOOCCLUSIVE BONE PAIN CRISIS.

Pain management as discussed.

Treat the cause [malaria, sepsis, dehydration].

Adequate hydration, taking care not to have a fluid overload [60mls/kg/24hrs or 3L per day].

Vital signs monitoring [patient placed on a monitor].

Respiratory Rate must be monitored.

If this ranges between 35 & 40 per minute, then patient must be moved to the intensive care unit.

SPO2 monitoring.

Ventilator support if spO2 is less than 95%.

PCV monitoring.

Haemoglobin Concentration must not be less than 9.5g/dL.

If there is severe anaemia of about 18% PCV, then, there must be RED BLOOD CELL TRANSFUSION till PCV becomes 27-28%.

Exchange blood transfusion is a better option for a refractory VOC [Vaso occlusive crisis] (under the watch of the haematology team!).

INTRAPARTUM CARE

Labour pain control gold standard is epidural analgesia, for vaginal delivery.

Pethidine must never be used to control labour pain because of the risk of seizure.

In places like Nigeria, where epidural analgesia is impossible because of the logistics and the cost implication, pentazocine has been the saving grace.

For a caesarean section, regional anaesthesia is the gold standard.

Induction of labour should be done by 38th week of gestation, except there is a contraindication or there's an obstetric indication for a caesarean section.

During labour, continuous intrapartum electronic foetal heart rate monitoring is recommended because of the increased risk of foetal distress.

In the event of increased foetal distress, then a caesarean section is indicated!

Patient must be well hydrated, but should not be overhydrated.

A fluid chart should be opened so that overhydration can be prevented.

Gold standard fluid during labour is normal saline (60mls/kg/24hrs or 3 litres daily).

Patient must be kept warm during labour.

PCV must be taken EVERY 2 HOURS.

Urinalysis must be done EVERY SINGLE TIME THE WOMAN VOIDS URINE to check for proteinuria and glucosuria (a pointer to preeclampsia and gestational diabetes respectively).

Vital signs which include the blood pressure, the temperature, the pulse rate, the respiratory rate and the pulse oximetry must be done EVERY HOUR.

The spleen and liver span must be done EVERY HOUR so that any acute sequestration crises can be caught early.

Patient delivery must involve a multidisciplinary team, which include a senior midwife and a senior anaesthetist, an haematologist with experience and profound interest in managing pregnant sickle cell patients and an obstetrician vast in managing high risk pregnancies.

The delivery must be taken in a tertiary health institution.

This institution must have INTENSIVE CARE UNIT FACILITIES.

Ideally, there should be a MONITOR so that any slight anomaly in vital signs can be noticed early and intercepted immediately.

When the pulse oximetry reading(spo2) becomes less than 95%, then the patient should be placed on facial oxygen.

If the spO2 reading does not improve, then the patient should be managed in the ICU (Intensive Care Unit).

A school of thought recommends oxygen administration from the onset of labour.

POSTPARTUM CARE

Immediate postpartum care involves managing in the labour ward for another 4 hours.

Perineal pad placement to monitor bleeding.

Vital signs, liver and spleen span measured EVERY HOUR.

PCV done every 2 HOUR.

Urinalysis done EVERY SINGLE TIME PATIENT VOIDS URINE.

Fluid management remains at 60mls/kg/hr or 3 litres daily.

Oral fluid intake should be encouraged.

Patient should be transferred to the postnatal ward from the labour ward after about 4 days if all parameters are normal and depending on the peculiarities of the case.

2 HOURLY PCV monitoring continues for another 24 hours.

It's then reduced to TWICE DAILY FOR ANOTHER 4 DAYS approximately (depending on the patient's peculiarities).

Vital signs, spleen and liver span monitoring to be also reduced (to EVERY 4 HOURS).

Urinalysis to be reduced to ONCE DAILY FOR ANOTHER 4 DAYS.

Vasoocclusive bone pain crisis, Urinary Tract Infection, Acute Chest Syndrome, pulmonary embolism, ischaemic stroke, Acute Anaemia (secondary to acute haemolytic crisis, splenic sequestration crisis, or aplastic crisis), are all common during the postpartum period, just like in the antenatal period.

These complications are managed the same way they were managed during antenatal care.

If baby was delivered through a Caesarean section, the mother must be on low molecular weight heparin during hospital stay and for 6 weeks after discharge, to prevent any risk of clot formation (thrombosis), and clot travelling to vital organs like the lungs and the brain (thromboembolic events: pulmonary embolism and ischaemic stroke).

If the baby was delivered through a vaginal delivery, the mother should be on low molecular weight heparin, during hospital stay too and for 1 week after discharge (for the same reason highlighted in 3. above).

For the same reasons highlighted in (3.) antithrombotic stockings are recommended in the puerperium, according to Royal College Of Gynaecologists Green-top Guidelines.

The mother must be well educated by the health care professionals about the risk of postpartum haemorrhage(bleeding and soaking of blood through more than one pad an hour or blood clots that's about the size of an egg or bigger); postpartum depression (thoughts of hurting oneself or the baby); postpartum leaking (urine leaking/urinary incontinence after birth)etc.

She must be informed about having a low threshold of visiting the hospital when she notices the first two signs. They are red flags!

She must also be educated about the immunization schedules for the newborn which she must comply with.

The need for contraception and family planning must also be emphasised, because the risks associated with pregnancy in sickle cell are quite much and can be fatal. The contraceptive options must be explained to her, so that she chooses what works best for her.

Some school of thoughts strongly recommends bilateral tubal ligation(BTL), especially after she already has two kids.

A solid support system must be available for domestic chores, caring for the woman and her baby.

Skin to skin contact, playing with the baby and not being separated(at any time) from him/her during the puerperium must be encouraged.

Newborn screening for sickle cell disease is a must especially if the mother and father are both carriers.

Adequate diet must be given to the mother, to replenish her, build her immunity and also compensate for breastfeeding.

The food items recommended include: eggs, beef, nuts and seeds, leafy greens, legumes (peanuts, beans, etc)whole wheat bread, brown rice, whole grains, salmons and other oily fish, fruits, ginger, almonds, adequate hydration (water).

The relatives of the new mother must be educated about the best practices in the care of the newborn and its mother; especially matters around adequate diet for the mother, exclusive breastfeeding for the child (6 months span), and umbilical cord care.

One of such best practice is that baby shouldn't be bathed until after 24hrs of delivery.

If possible, there should be policies put in place by the government to facilitate better support in the workplace for the new mother and her baby.

Preterm babies and low birth weight babies must be administered special care.

The mother must be educated thoroughly about the following signs in their babies, and the need to seek emergency care immediately must be emphasised. These signs are not peculiar to just sickle cell patients who just had a baby: when the baby stops feeding well, begins to convulse, breath rapidly (≥ 60 cycles per minute), begins to have severe chest in-drawing, ceases to have spontaneous movements, has a fever (temperature ≥ 37.5 °C), a low body temperature (temperature < 35.5 °C), has any jaundice in first 24 hours of life, or yellow palms and soles at any age.

These signs are red flags and must not be taken for granted!

Apart from postpartum haemorrhage and postpartum depression, there are other red flags to also look out for in the sickle cell patient who just delivered. These red flags are not peculiar to only sickle cell mothers.

They include: headaches not responding to analgesics or with affected vision, obstructed breathing/shortness of breath/increased rate of breathing, incision wounds that would not heal, a fever($\geq 38^0$c), chest pain, vaginal discharge with very foul odour, pain, warmth, swelling and redness at the calf region, seizures etc.

Diclofenac and other Nonsteroidal Anti-inflammatory Drugs can be taken for pain relief during breastfeeding; they're not contraindicated by breastfeeding.

CHAPTER 4

BONUSES:

The following are articles that I wrote, in the course of marketing my books and event management business.

They are extremely relevant to both genders in the sickle cell community; a few are however specific to the pregnant woman; not just the pregnant sickle cell patient.

Some of this information was already emphasised earlier in this book though.

1.NAIRA MARLEY AND MOHBAD SAGA :

"Mohbad IS LIKELY to have been killed by drug overdose secondary to ADDICTION ", a Consultant Psychiatrist in the University College Hospital, Ibadan, reported.

Many sickle cell patients in Nigeria have found themselves in this kind of tragic state(ADDICTION) because of ignorance, mismanagement by healthcare professionals, increased cost of booking a doctor's appointment, absence of or unaffordable cost of advanced treatment options in Nigeria, self-medication, and many more.

ADDICTION VS PSEUDO-ADDICTION VS DEPENDENCY

ADDICTION in sickle cell disease is characterised by:

A. A compulsive intake of drug despite knowledge of its adverse effects.

B. Registration with multiple hospitals to have increased access to narcotics.

C. Using different names, dates of birth and identities in order to give the impression it's a different individual in need of the opioids.

D. Forgery of doctors' signatures.

E. Selling of properties to purchase narcotics.

F. Insistence on the increment of dosage and frequency of opioid administration and neglecting other treatment options.

G. Refusal to allow tapering down of the opioids.

H. Sharing of opioid analgesics among sickle cell patients on hospital admission.

PSEUDOADDICTION is the same except for the fact that PAIN IS TRULY AND HONESTLY NOT CONTROLLED.

DEPENDENCE is when a patient needs a higher dose of opioid to achieve the same analgesic effect.

Addiction always presents with dependence but dependence is not addiction but also a serious side effect of opioid analgesics.

Addiction is a great concern and issue among sickle cell patients in Nigeria, especially to the notorious pentazocine.

TREATING PAIN IN SICKLE CELL DISEASE

There are two types of pain in sickle cell: chronic pain and acute pain. The two, however can occur at the same time.

In severity, it's classified into mild, moderate and severe.

Acute pain is caused majorly by Vaso-occlusive bone pain crisis.

Chronic pain is caused majorly by AVN(Avascular Necrosis of the hip joint), sickle cell leg ulcers and chronic osteomyelitis.

The management (treatment) of pain is based on the cause, the type, the severity and whether a patient is opioid-tolerant or opioid-naive.

Sickle cell nephropathy (Kidney issues), asthmatic exacerbation, peptic ulcer disease, and perforation from a peptic ulcer are side effects that can come from use(long term or short term) of NSAIDS(diclofenac, Ibuprofen etc) as well.

It is therefore important to up our game in the management of pain in sickle cell disease.

EFFECTIVE PAIN MANAGEMENT IN SICKLE CELL DISEASE [WITH EMPHASIS ON PREVENTING ADDICTION, PSEUDO-ADDICTION AND DEPENDENCE IN SICKLE CELL DISEASE]

1. TREAT THE CAUSE of the pain, not just the pain symptom. Malaria and sepsis ("infection in the blood") are the major cause of acute pain in sickle cell anaemia.

Chronic pain is caused majorly by AVN(Avascular Necrosis) of the hip and some other joints, sickle cell leg ulcers and chronic osteomyelitis.

2. Malaria prophylaxis to prevent pain recurrence from malaria.

3. Acute pain from bone infarction should be treated with NSAIDS, if the patient is not a known peptic ulcer disease(PUD), asthmatic nor a nephropathy patient. This is because bone pain in sickle-cell is inflammatory in nature.

4. Pain physicians should be able to distinguish between mild, moderate and severe pain so they can know what moment to step up to strong opioids for their patients.

5. Differential diagnosis of pain in sickle cell disease must not always be sickle cell related (vaso-occlusive crisis etc).

Osteoarthritis, rheumatoid arthritis, tuberculous arthritis, and many more can happen in sickle cell patients too.

Thinking outside this box of sickle cell-related pain helps to discover early and treat other possible causes of pain effectively; therefore long-term opioid analgesic use is limited.

Angina pectoris (from a heart disease), Neuralgias, Neuropathies, psychiatric conditions and many more can present with pain too, which is USUALLY NOT sickle cell related.

6. Chest pain can be a symptom of pulmonary embolism, fat embolism syndrome and acute chest syndrome; the causes must be treated not just the symptom. THESE ARE EMERGENCIES.

7. Depression is a cause of chronic pain which doesn't respond to regular analgesics. I had this for several months until I was placed on antidepressants.

8. Opioids (Morphine, Hydromorphone, Diamorphine, Dihydrocodeine, pethidine and other opioids), if indispensable, should be combined with other analgesics which are not opioids, so that there can be a synergistic effect and reduced need to increase opioid dosage and frequency.

9. Taking history of the last opioid administration, opioid type and dosage, to know if a patient is opioid-tolerant or opioid-naive.

10. Cannabidiol is a less addictive analgesic, but research is still ongoing for its safety.

11. Health care professionals must be able to distinguish between addiction, pseudo-addiction and dependence, so that they can adequately manage pain and refer patients who need a psychiatric intervention as soon as possible.

12. Nerve block for chronic pain like AVN (with or without opioids).

13. Lidocaine patch for leg ulcers.

14. Orthopaedic interventions (e.g. devices to limit exertion of load on joints affected by AVN).

15. Orthopaedic surgery for AVN; although total hip replacement surgery is only indicated if pain becomes completely unbearable.

16. Physiotherapy.

17. Massage.

18. Cognitive behavioural therapy to help patients develop coping mechanisms for chronic pain.

19. Reduced health care cost [BY THE GOVERNMENT] so that patients will prefer to see a doctor for their prescription and other treatment options for pain, rather than cutting corners to get opioid analgesics.

20. GOVERNMENT should put in place and make affordable advanced pain management options; they should also sponsor research projects on better pain management drugs and methods.

21. Increased empathy for sickle cell patients. Our pains heal faster when we don't have psychological issues.

22. Restoration of broken homes and relationships which can trigger and worsen pain episodes. Some addicts in the sickle cell community were found to be victims of the former. I personally was tempted to increase co-codamol dosage when I had a pain episode during a relationship crisis I recently called off.

23. Removing any other issues that could constitute psychological imbalance.

24. Health care professionals should try and believe our report of pain to prevent pseudo-addiction.

25. Pharmacists and pharmacy stores should try and do better by giving opioids only on prescription.

26. To prevent withdrawal symptoms seen in opioid dependence, tapering opioid analgesics down after pain relief is compulsory!

27. Continuous research on acute and chronic pain management in sickle cell disease.

28. Patients should try and open up if they see any signs of addiction which I wrote above.

29. Doctors, nurses and other healthcare professionals must not be judgemental and must earn/gain the trust of their addict patients; To feel well and recover speedily, patients should banish the feelings of guilt and condemnation which are part and parcel of addiction.

You need to know what God says about addicts. I wrote them in my books.

30. Get my books about pain management(treatment), addiction prevention and management (treatment) in sickle cell disease, what God says about addicts, and the list of other addictive drugs.

To get this book, kindly reply, BOOK , using this WhatsApp number:

https://wa.me/2348020878841

2. THE CURE TO SICKLE CELL DISEASE: BONE MARROW TRANSPLANT!

SICKLE CELL AND THE GOSPEL; ANY RELATIONSHIP?

BLOOD TRANSFUSION VS EXCHANGE BLOOD TRANSFUSION VS BONE MARROW TRANSPLANT; ANY DIFFERENCE?

Once upon a time, there lived a man who had and still has a burning love for the world.

He offered life to the first man(Adam) but the man chose death over life.

This didn't change his reckless love towards this man and several generations that came after him.

Several parables of the ultimate redemption plan were set in place:

Sometimes, the blood of bulls, goats and calves will be used as a cleansing measure for the sins of these people.

At the same time, a scapegoat receives the sins of these people through a priest who lays his hands on the goat to transfer the sins of the people; there was an EXCHANGE and the goat is led into a journey of no return (DESTRUCTION), so that the sins of the people can be punished. (Leviticus 16:20-22)

The blood of the bulls, goats and calves; and this particular scapegoat was not sufficient to provide a ONCE AND FOR ALL atonement for sins; therefore, these rituals were done every year(repeatedly).

After so many years of repeated sacrifices, the promise about the ultimate atonement came to pass.

This man who has this burning love for the world, came to the world by himself.

His blood (life) was shed just like those of the bulls, goats and calves.

He received the sins of the world just like the scape goat and offers the world LIFE and RIGHTEOUSNESS (A PHENOMENAL EXCHANGE).

The difference between His sacrifices and those of the animals earlier used is:

1. His sacrifice was a one time/ once and for all atonement that is POTENT TILL ETERNITY.(Hebrews 9:12-14; Hebrews 10:4,12,14)

2. This sacrifice also inputs the Life of God/the Spirit of God into anyone that believes.(John 3:16; Ephesians 1:13)

The blood of bulls, goats and calves; and the scape goat atonement was not sufficient to give the Eternal Life of God/ His Spirit to any of the people whose sins were being washed.

HOW DOES THIS STORY RELATE TO SICKLE CELL?

THE BULLS', GOATS', AND CALVES' BLOOD which is needed to be sprinkled every now and then, is what blood transfusion looks like in reality.

Physically and spiritually, blood represents life. (Leviticus 17:11)

In sickle cell disease, if blood transfusion is not done in some cases, then the patient will definitely die!

The scapegoat upon whom the sins of the people was exchanged is what EXCHAGE BLOOD TRANSFUSION sounds like.

The unhealthy blood is taken and EXCHANGED FOR THE HEALTHY ONE ; The unhealthy blood is discarded, just like the scape goat was destroyed.

Exchange blood transfusion and regular blood transfusion are used to temporarily treat some complications and crises in sickle cell disease!

Unfortunately, that you have had a blood transfusion or an exchange blood transfusion before does not mean you won't have complications/crises that'd require you to have another one!

So, exactly how these bull, goat, calf and scapegoat sacrifices gets perpetually repeated; so it can be for blood transfusion and exchange blood transfusion.

However, Bone Marrow Transplant (BMT) involves harvesting that particular tissue that creates life(blood) and getting this into the patient's body.

Like this sacrificial man, who laid down his life, a sibling offers to give a sickle cell patient his/her bone marrow.

Now, the sickle cell patient has the life generator, like every believer has the holy ghost; the Life of God that never dies!

The sickle cell patients, after bone marrow transplant can offer to share part of his blood(life), with another individual at the point of death; just like every believer can give the life of God in them by sharing the gospel with an unbeliever!

So, Bone Marrow Transplant(BMT) is a game changer in sickle cell disease; just like the gospel of Christ is the ultimate, irreversible, everlasting, once and for all and the permanent atonement for sins!

Copyright held by Dr. Agboola Emmanuel Tobiloba.

An addendum to TALES AND PARABLES DEMYSTIFYING THE TRUTHS AND MYTHS OF SICKLE CELL DISEASE

HARDCOPIES of my books now available including: MY JOURNEY FROM PAIN TO POWER WITH 24 COMPLICATIONS OF SICKLE CELL ANAEMIA.

I partner with an organization in India who offers first class services for bone marrow transplant.

Reply BMT to my WhatsApp link below to know how you can access this opportunity at an affordable rate.

Reply HARD to my WhatsApp link below to order for your hard copies now!

https://wa.me/2348020878841

Permission to share is granted!

3.ISRAEL AND PALESTINE are not the only locations where there are bomb blasts.

I got one in a WhatsApp group and my phone almost caught fire:

"FOLIC ACID IS NOT IMPORTANT IN SICKLE CELL DISEASE MANAGEMENT", A SICKLE CELL PATIENT SAID!

I retorted:

"Sickle cell is a chronic illness characterised by chronic anaemia which predisposes the sickle cell patient to ventricular hypertrophy.

Folic acid is basic and you must not toy with it.

Old age cometh soon, when you shall see why your doctors recommend folic acid!

Read parable of the lame man's hands and legs in my book and you'll understand what hypertrophy of the heart muscles(ventricle) is.

The heart is straining itself to supply you enough oxygen because of the chronic anaemic state in a sickle cell patient.

Folic acid is meant to make more red blood cells so that more haemoglobin will be available to supply more oxygen around your body.

When there is anaemia, the cells are deprived of oxygen and the heart has to be overworked to compensate for this.

Folic acid produces more red blood cells that carry more haemoglobin; which helps to increase oxygen supply to the tissues; consequently reducing the tension and the compensatory work load on the heart.

Sickle cell is not just about acute presentations(pain etc).

You are gradually laying your bed where you're going to sleep in years to come (old age).

Multiple organ failure can result from chronic hypoxia too(a result of chronic anaemia).

In hypertension, you may feel well until you come down with a stroke or blindness (hypertensive retinopathy).

So, it's not about feeling well.

You may feel well, but investigations and doctors' examinations tell you that you are not well!

Feeling well is not a yardstick that a sickle cell patient is well!

And that's why regular check ups are important!

In pregnancy too, folic acid prevents you from having a baby whose brain and spinal cord won't be completely enveloped by the skull and the spinal column(back bone) respectively.

The exposure of the spinal cord and the brain with other related birth defects is what we call NEURAL TUBE DEFECTS(NTDs).

If you will joke with your heart and your vital organs, don't joke with your unborn child!

Excerpt from the book "SICKLE CELL UNMARKED".

To have more insights about treating and managing a sickle cell child or adult, kindly message me to get a copy each of my two other books on sickle cell disease:

https://wa.me/2348020878841

4. ATIKU ABUBAKAR'S state (Adamawa, Nigeria) , there lived a farmer, who was very rich, but not so intelligent.

This farmer used mechanised irrigation for his large-scale farming, especially during the Harmattan season. He leveraged on the expertise of an Agricultural Engineer.

Unfortunately, debris deposits (algae, bacterial slime, precipitates, construction debris, and sediment) came along with the water occasionally.

Each time this happened, the terminal pipes with smaller diameters got blocked by those deposits.

Consequently, there was cessation of water supply to the plants. The plants then began to wither, starting from the leaves (and other shoot systems).

The water needed to dissolve and take nutrients to the plant tissues had been cut off.

The rich farmer had fired the Agricultural Engineer, because he thought his services were no longer needed.

Therefore, there was no one to monitor and maintain the irrigation system. Eventually, the whole plantation withered off completely!

HOW DOES THIS STORY RELATE TO SICKLE CELL ANAEMIA?

A high percentage of symptoms, clinical features and complications that has ever been recorded about Sickle Cell Disease has the same analogy with the just-concluded story.

There are pipes (arteries) that supply blood to all organs and tissues in humans.

In Sickle Cell Anaemia, the red blood cells, under certain adverse conditions, turn into the shape of a SICKLE, clump together and block the terminal pipes (capillaries).

Because Oxygen is carried by this blood to our organs through these pipes; blockage results in hypoxia (reduced tissue oxygen).

The hypoxia causes injury to the tissues affected, just like the plant story narrated above.

When the blockage of blood supply becomes repeated, or is severe enough, the injury proceeds to "withering" of the organs affected (they begin to "wither" like the plants described above).

In human pathology however, this " WITHERING " is what we doctors call NECROSIS .

The block of blood supply is what we call ISCHAEMIA.

When NECROSIS happens because of ISCHAEMIA, it's called INFARCTION.

MORAL OF THE STORY:

Water/hydration is indispensable in the long term management of sickle cell disease and in the prevention of most crises and complications of the disease.

Don't fire your irrigation engineer !

Excerpt from the book, " SICKLE CELL UNMASKED "

[THE PARABLE OF THE FOOLISH FARMER: ONE OF THE MANY INTERESTING TALES AND PARABLES IN THE BOOK, DEMYSTIFYING THE TRUTHS AND MYTHS OF SICKLE CELL DISEASE].

To see the end of this story and more stories used to illustrate and simplify the medical terms of sickle cell, message me now to get my two other books containing these stories:

https://wa.me/2348020878841

5. EMERGENCY!

SICKLE CELL DISEASE EMERGENCIES AND MORE:

A. SICKLE CELL RETINOPATHY makes some sickle cell patients lose their sights.

This is more common with Haemoglobin SC patients than Haemoglobin SS.

PREVENTING VISION LOSS IN SICKLE CELL DISEASE

1. Regular eye examination with an ophthalmologist and

2. Hydroxyurea

B. ISCHAEMIC STROKE

Transcranial Doppler Ultrasound Scan is a must for paediatric Sickle Cell patients.

This scan catches early any imminent ischaemic STROKE, which is very common in paediatric sickle cell patients.

A stroke is an emergency too, whether in sickle cell or hypertension:

You can diagnose a stroke using the acronym: F.A.S.T

F.........Face drooping
A.........Arm weakness
S.........Speech difficulty
T..........Time to bolt to the EMERGENCY ROOM

Stroke is irreversible.

The earlier your patient gets to the hospital the better.

Take patient to a sophisticated hospital (which would not need you to have a referral)

C. CHEST PAIN

Chest pain in sickle cell disease is an emergency!

It could be a sign of:

1. Pulmonary embolism
2. Fat embolism syndrome
3. Acute chest syndrome

All three can take a life in minutes!

D. Iron-containing multivitamins are contraindicated in(SHOULD NOT BE GIVEN TO) sickle cell patients.

The rapid rate of haemolysis (red blood cell destruction/breakdown) in sickle-cell patients makes our system laden with iron.

This iron laden in our system can be reused when erythropoiesis (red blood cell production) takes place.

If additional iron is given, then iron overload sets in.

A good example of multivitamin that doesn't contain iron is ASTYMIN.

ASTYFER CONTAINS IRON PLEASE!

It is logical that we have more than enough iron, since iron constitutes the haemoglobin in red blood cells!

To get more information about the management of sickle cell disease (in children, women [pregnant and non-pregnant], in psychiatry etc), these books are strongly recommended.

Contact Dr. Agboola Emmanuel now to get your copies immediately:

https://wa.me/2348020878841

6.SICKLE CELL CHILD CARE

VACCINES AND IMMUNISATIONS

1. At 2-3 months Penicillin V must be commenced and given twice daily.

2. If child is allergic (reacts adversely) to Penicillins, Erythromycin should be given instead.

3. Meningococcal vaccine.

4. Pneumococcal Vaccine.

5. After 6 months, a child must have a booster dose of the Pneumococcal Vaccine.

6. Haemophilus Influenza type B Vaccine (HIB vaccine).

7. All other immunisations recommended for every other child.

ROUTINE DRUGS AND SUPPLEMENTS

1. FOLIC ACID.

2. The Malaria Prophylactic (medication preventing malaria) is PROGUANIL (50mg-100mg daily depending on age and weight).

3. HYDROXYUREA, depending on your child's level of Foetal Haemoglobin and severity of complications and crises.

Kindly note that not all patients respond satisfactorily to Hydroxyurea; most patients do though.

4. Astymin, Vitamin C and Vitamin B Complex are not out of place, but are not routinely prescribed (in the University College Hospital, Ibadan for example).

CARE RESPONSIBILITIES ON THE PARENTS (MOTHER ESPECIALLY)

1. Routine Spleen Palpation to catch enlargement early. Spleen enlargement could be a sign of these three life-threatening conditions: ACUTE SPLENIC SEQUESTRATION CRISIS, SPLENOMEGALY OR HYPERSPLENISM.

The mother should know the approximate size of the spleen (located at the left upper quadrant of the abdomen) and this should enable her detect very fast any enlargement.

2. Have a THERMOMETER at home and measure your child's TEMPERATURE as often as possible. A fever symptom (high temperature) in your child must get you and

your child to the nearest Emergency Room (Hospital) at the speed of light.

3. Don't miss doctors' appointments even if your child is not ill.

4. Keep your child warm during cold weather.

5. Hydrate them properly (Give them enough water) always, especially during the dry and hot weather.

6. You as a parent should know that your Sickle Cell child is healthy for most of the period or time; they fall ill during just a small fraction of their lifetime and therefore not more disadvantaged than their counterparts, peers or age group!

7. A VASOOCCLUSIVE BONE PAIN CRISIS which is MILD and which does not come with a FEVER can be managed at home with an analgesic like Ibuprofen. If there is a fever or if bone pain worsens or doesn't resolve, please head to the hospital at the speed of light!

THE COMPULSORY INVESTIGATION TO BE DONE EVERY 12 MONTHS BETWEEN AGE 2 YEARS AND 16 YEARS!

TRANSCRANIAL DOPPLER ULTRASOUND SCAN(TCD): This is an investigation that is used to check for the velocity (speed) of blood flow in the brain.

If the speed goes above 200 centimetres per second, then a STROKE is almost definitely around the corner, and management is commenced immediately!

To learn more about the management of sickle cell disease, kindly message me to get my two other books on sickle cell disease:

https://wa.me/2348020878841

7. DEPRESSION IS COMMON AMONG SICKLE CELL PATIENTS.

PSYCHOTHERAPY TIPS AND OTHER MEASURES FOR SICKLE CELL PATIENTS

(EXCERPTS FROM MY TWO BOOKS: SICKLE CELL UNMASKED AND SHINING THROUGH THE DARK TUNNEL)

1. DON'T LIVE ALONE:

Emergencies can happen anytime.

At such times, you will need some support to get to the hospital!

2. CRY FOR HELP AS OFTEN AS IT BECOMES OVERWHELMING:

Do not suffer in silence in the name of FAITH.

Faith has its place, but your Haematologists, Psychotherapists and Psychiatrists have their place too.

It is absolutely normal to be depressed in the sickle cell journey.

I have been there and I contemplated suicide.

Before things go out of hand and become unsalvageable,

please reach out for urgent help from your specialists, your family and your friends.

As a matter of fact approximately 35.2% of adult sickle cell patients have been diagnosed at least once, with depression.

29% of us have had suicidal thoughts at one point or the other in our lifetime!

About 8% of us actually advanced to ATTEMPT SUICIDE.

So, before it reaches thinking suicide at all, please kindly reach out for help!

3. IF YOU FEEL LIKE CRYING, PLEASE CRY, AND DON'T HESITATE TO GET BACK UP QUICKLY:

Sometimes, crying is therapeutic and relieves you of those bad emotions and burden.

When you cry, don't stay too long there.

Pick up yourself and move on again!

4. CATCH AT LEAST 8 HOURS SLEEP A DAY.

5. DON'T BUILD YOUR WORLD AROUND ANYONE:

This has tremendously damaged my mental and emotional health.

Thank God, my life didn't go in exchange!

Please kindly note that you need help.

But if this help ain't forthcoming, do not let it get at you.

6. MAKE PLENTY OF FRIENDS:

This will prevent you from being seen as a liability by the few ones you have.

By making plenty friends, you'll share your burdens and pains into lighter pieces, that's hardly felt by each of your friends.

7. LET YOUR FRIENDS KNOW THAT YOU ARE ON HOSPITAL ADMISSION:

I learnt this the hard way.

It was in my final year that I realised that I have not carried anyone along as a friend,

through my sickle cell journey in the University of Ibadan.

I had a heartbreak at this time, was commenced on ANTITUBERCULOSIS, ANTIDEPRESSANTS, ANTI-INSOMNIA, ANTIBIOTICS, and ANALGESICS all at the same time; almost failed my final year resit exams because of the heartbreak.

Heartbreaks reveal nakedness and emptiness; especially when you don't have backup friends.

Having friends (who you like and who really cares about you) around you on your hospital bed or admission gives you that euphoric sensation and helps you heal faster.

Also, I learnt in a hard way that I was supposed to detach myself from my parents and survive on the shoulders of multiple friends as I attained adulthood.

You should try to practice this too, because you won't stay forever with your parents!

8. BELONG TO SICKLE CELL SUPPORT GROUPS AND OTHER EDIFYING GROUPS:

Iron sharpens iron!

It is dangerous to be a lone ranger.

Preys that fall out of the herd are the most susceptible to being killed by the predator.

The essence of a herd or a pack of animals is to reinforce each others' strength.

Once one of them falls out, and doesn't come back as soon as possible, then, it's gone forever!

A bunch of brooms is really difficult to get broken.

That's the essence of a group.

Belonging to groups is especially important if depression has set in!

9. HAVE A SICKLE CELL WARRIOR THAT YOU LOOK UP TO :

Tell these folks who are ahead of you to tell you how they overcame those challenges.

Their stories alone can spark you up, energise you and strengthen you!

10: HAVE A FIRM GRIP ON GOD'S WORD.

Please, I'd recommend that you get my other book:

SHINING THROUGH THE DARK TUNNEL.

In the book, I explained how my self-esteem and self-worth were restored through aggressively feeding on MY IDENTITIES IN CHRIST.

I also explained how I almost ran mad, simply because I THOUGHT MY JUSTIFICATION AND RIGHTEOUSNESS WAS TO BE EARNED BY MY GOOD WORKS.

I was tremendously tormented with the fear of going to hell, until I met a good teacher who put me through.

The teacher was able to prove to me through tons of bible passages that,

EVERLASTING SALVATION, REDEMPTION AND FORGIVENESS OF SINS ONLY COME TO A MAN AFTER HE BELIEVES AND CONFESSES THAT JESUS CHRIST DIED, WAS BURIED AND WAS RESURRECTED FOR THAT INDIVIDUAL'S FORGIVENESS.

In-depth and extremely thorough knowledge that I got from this teacher healed my insanity and madness.

I could think straight again, with no torments of the fear of hell anymore!

That's what knowledge in God's word can do.

Sickle cell has succeeded in giving many of its victims low self-esteem and inferiority complex.

I wasn't exempted!

I redefined myself using God's word.

Details of this redefinition and identity discovery is in the book:

SHINING THROUGH THE DARK TUNNEL.

You'll get tremendous and incredible value for your money, I promise you this!

11. THE PLACE OF FAITH:

Faith carried me through the most part of my journey especially when all efforts to curb obsessive compulsive disorder(OCD) episodes and depression proved abortive.

You can cry to God, say a word of prayer.

You may want to pray the aggressive way.

I've done all these before!

It was an intense agony then, battling depression and OCD.

Faith and prayers connected me miraculously to the doctors that prescribed the breakthrough drugs for my mental health!

12. REPLACE YOUR WORRIES WITH MEDITATION:

Worries take you nowhere!

So, replace those negative thoughts with God's opinion and assertions about you:

A. You are forgiven because you have believed Jesus' death, burial and resurrection as a sacrifice for your sins,

(if you have never believed this information before now, you need to make that decision right now!!!)

B. You are healed,

C. You are justified

D. You're not condemned

E. You're the head and not the tail ………

My second book talks extensively about these bible passages and I must tell you that tremendous value awaits you in that book.

So, instead of giving worry a chance, please kindly think (meditate) on the precious names and identities that God has lovingly named you!

Whatever you think about, you bring about!

Thoughts are things!

So, act accordingly!

13. PUT GOD'S WORDS ON YOUR LIPS:

The same things that you meditate on, let them be spoken out of your mouth!

It's called confession of faith!

The book of Mark says if you tell a mountain to move from here to the other side, you shall absolutely have what you have said.

So, speak out what you want over and about your life!

14. DARE TO SET GOALS THAT ARE TREMENDOUSLY MORE GIGANTIC THAN YOU ARE:

These goals have the capacity to keep your eyes off your present challenges as a sickle cell warrior.

GIGANTIC GOALS have powerful "magnetic fields" that irresistibly force you towards themselves, regardless of how low or down you have gone.

They have the capacity to make you always rise again in tireless pursuit of those dreams!

15. HAVE A TO-DO LIST FOR EVERY SINGLE DAY:

A To-do list helps you break down your gigantic goals into bits and pieces.

Having something already outlined for you to do everyday makes you have exciting reasons to wake up to life everyday!

16. BE CONSISTENTLY, PERSISTENTLY, HABITUALLY AND DELIBERATELY GRATEFUL:

Counting your blessings gives you that sense of immense joy and fulfilment.

Counting your blessings makes you see clearly how strong you have been, how much you have achieved, how dogged, resilient and rugged you have been and how purposeful and laser-focused you have been.

The more you count, the more amazed and dazed you become.

Seeing clearly what you have achieved so far motivates you to want to do more!

17. DISCOVER YOURSELF:

Sickle cell gave me two lemons which I turned into lemonades.

In Sickle Cell Anaemia, puberty is either reached late, or some secondary sexual characteristics become absent.

Most sickle cell patients in developing countries,

including the adult ones look far younger than their age and they tend to be disrespected for this.

I've had my fair share, but it became a prominent compliment that I receive at least every 60 days.

My patients and other acquaintances are confused how a young person like me could find his way into a profession as noble as this.

This makes me very motivated to even perform better.

At puberty, I couldn't attain the baritone voice characteristic of an adolescent or the adult male gender.

Each time I speak over the phone with somebody for the first time, they always assume that it's a lady speaking.

This has never been embarrassing to me, rather I find it really amusing that nobody ever gets my gender correctly by just listening to my voice.

To cap it all off, I sing beautifully well with this same voice, that even ladies covet the voice!!!

I noticed that I am also very empathetic with my patients.

This empathy is partly because of the tenets of the profession and most importantly, because I KNOW WHAT PAIN FEELS LIKE.

So, I'm very gentle with my patients.

All these three qualities make me feel good about myself, let me know how much lives I've impacted, and how much the blessings of God is upon me!

Why these stories?

It's just to let you realise that there's something unique and very different about you.

Look inwards and bring them out.

Unleash them!

Discovering your hidden potentials and unique abilities makes you find tremendously irresistible reasons to wake up each day happily and stay alive to impact others with these unique elements in you.

You may want to reach me on this line, so we can talk about fulfilling purpose:

https://wa.me/2348020878841

This is a topic whose teachings are sufficient enough to write another book!

18. REACH OUT TO THOSE WHO ARE STRUGGLING ON THE SAME ROAD YOU TRIUMPHANTLY JOURNEYED THROUGH:

This brings tremendous fulfilment!

Seeing those you helped after they're out of the challenges is such a thrilling experience.

I'm so fulfilled helping you through this journey through my two books and my sickle cell groups.

Wouldn't you want that kind of fulfilment?

19. FIND YOUR PASSION:

Finding your passion makes work become play for you.

You don't get exhausted easily if your work is a field you are in love with!

20. REWARD YOURSELF:

Anytime you conquer a task or any seemingly difficult situation, reward yourself.

At every single bit of success too, please do the same.

Rewarding yourself motivates you to do more and prevents you from being worn out easily!

I DRAW THE CURTAIN HERE!

To get more tips about how to weather the storms of(survive and thrive in) sickle cell disease, please kindly message me through my WhatsApp link,

https://wa.me/2348020878841 ,

and type BOOK to buy a copy each of my two books, containing these information.

8. PREGNANT SICKLE CELL PATIENT.

First off, I deliberately delayed my Christmas and New Year wishes to you so that this article will not be lost in the multitude of other messages you received as Christmas and New Year wishes.

Kindly remember the essence of Christmas:

Jesus came to save the world (including you and I) from their sins and everlasting destruction in hell by:

1. dying

2. being buried; and most importantly:

3. being raised from the dead on the third day.

This salvation can only be received by simply believing the three events listed and the information above.

This salvation is permanent and irreversible.

That said, Merry Christmas and Happy New Year in arrears!!!

Now, we rush into very important points to be noted about the peculiarities (including the dos and don'ts) of,

PREGNANCY IN A SICKLE CELL PATIENT.

1. MEDICATIONS IN PREGNANT SICKLE CELL DISEASE PATIENTS; DATES OF COMMENCEMENT AND DISCONTINUATION.

A. HYDROXYUREA (one of the medications used in managing Sickle Cell Disease) is known for being teratogenic(cause malformation in the baby in the womb).

HYDROXYUREA must be stopped 3 MONTHS before pregnancy!

B. Some ANTIHYPERTENSIVES (blood pressure medications) too,

(Angiotensin Converting Enzyme Inhibitors [benazepril captopril, enalapril, fosinopril, lisinopril, moexipril, perindopril, quinapril, ramipril, trandolapril etc],

& Angiotensin Receptor Blockers [irbesartan, valsartan, losartan, candesartan, etc]), must be discontinued,

because they are teratogenic (cause birth defects/malformations) and fetotoxic (can poison the foetus or embryo).

C. ANTIFOLATE ANTICONVULSANTS (drugs used to treat seizures) also must be discontinued (3 months before pregnancy) to prevent Neural Tube Defects.

D. AMINOGLYCOSIDES (E.G GENTAMICIN etc) AND TETRACYCLINE SHOULD NOT BE TAKEN BY A PREGNANT WOMAN:

The former are antibiotics that cause nephrotoxicity and ototoxicity (poisoning to the kidneys and the ears respectively) in the foetus.

The latter is an antibiotic that cause teeth discoloration in the foetus.

The long list of drugs that shouldn't be taken in pregnancy is not within the scope of this article.... smiles.

My book will let you know more!

2. IRON SUPPLEMENT VERSUS FOLIC ACID:

Iron Deficiency is the commonest cause of anaemia in pregnancy!

Iron overload is of a great concern in Sickle Cell Disease, because we have a load of store of iron in our bodies,

(secondary to inability of some iron to get excreted, the strikingly rapid rate of red blood cell destruction and repeated blood transfusions).

There's a kit used to assess Iron Deficiency.

It checks for the SERUM FERRITIN LEVEL.
This kit is not readily available in some parts of the world!

In these parts of the world, microcytosis on microscopy is the only available marker for Iron Deficiency.

There are now two types of anaemia that the pregnant SCD patient must deal with:

a. Sickle Cell Anaemia.

b. Iron Deficiency Anaemia.

Folate (Folic Acid) deficiency during the few months before pregnancy is strongly associated with Neural Tube Defects:

i. Spinal Bifida Occulta

ii. Anencephaly

iii. Myelomeningocele

iv. Encephalocele

v. Meningocele... etc

Iron Deficiency Anaemia is one of the most common causes of death in pregnant women!

SO, WHAT DO WE DO?

There was a compromise reached regarding Iron Overload vs Supplemental Iron in Pregnant SCD Patients, which I would subscribe to:

a. If there have been recent episodes of recurrent blood transfusions, then Iron should not be given.

b. If there have never been recurrent blood transfusions and the SCD Patient is confirmed to have Iron Deficiency, then, it is safe to give Iron Supplement

(Fersolate is one of the brands of medications used to supplement Iron in pregnant women).

c. For Folic Acid, routine Folic Acid for the mother must be taken for her own health.

d. If she is compliant with it, there would have been enough Folic Acid in her system to prevent the above-listed Neural Tube Defects,

(Folic Acid must be commenced 3 months before pregnancy).

Kindly note that Neural Tube Defects are defects that cause malformations in the spinal cord, the spinal column, the brain and the skull.

Extra dosage of Folic Acid is not needed for a Pregnant SCD Patient, if she has been compliant with her routine Folate.

Simply put, routine Folic Acid dosage in Pregnant SCD Patients is not increased because of their new state: pregnancy.

Kindly note that a history of having a child with Neural Tube Defects and a medical history of Diabetes Mellitus also predispose a pregnant woman to having a child with Neural Tube Defects.

To know more about the management of sickle cell disease (in a pregnant woman, in a child, in an adult, in a female patient etc),

kindly reach out to me on WhatsApp through this link:

https://wa.me/2348020878841 ,

and type PREGNANT to BUY a copy of my book which contains these details.

I love you now, and always !

9. WASTED LIFE CAUSED BY CARELESSNESS BEFORE, DURING AND AFTER PREGNANCY; DAMAGE COULD BE IRREVERSIBLE AND COULD COST YOU MORE THAN $1,000,000!

THAT UNBORN CHILD AND WIFE OF YOURS WILL THANK YOU FOR THESE; A LETTER TO YOU AND YOUR WIFE!

I hold the copyright to these information. Not copied nor pasted from anywhere. This is not a broadcast either; They were specifically typed out for you in two midnights!

So, I have a couple of clients whose weddings we'd be managing between August 2023 and April 2024.

Tons of outstanding offers/bonuses that no other wedding planner can possibly have on their list settled on my heart.

One of such bonuses is FREE PHYSICAL CONSULTATION [WITHIN THE FIRST THREE MONTHS OF PREGNANCY] WITH AN OBSTETRICIAN!

This is absolutely mouth-gaping; I can bet no wedding planner will prepare you ahead of your pregnancy!

I have 21 solid points to give to you right now, just like I shared with these couples (clients) of mine!

Like I said, ignorance about these facts can cost you a life and the destiny of the child in your womb (that's absolutely more than 1 million United States Dollars.)

LET'S SHOOT:

23 THINGS TO DO FOR YOUR UNBORN CHILD & YOUR WIFE TO SURVIVE AND BE IN PERFECT HEALTH; A LETTER TO YOUR WIFE!

A. FOLIC ACID MUST BE COMMENCED 3 MONTHS before pregnancy [or taken regularly by women of child-bearing age] to prevent Neural Tube Defects (defects affecting the brain, the skull, the spinal cord and the back bone).

B. POSTPARTUM HAEMORHAGE IS THE MAJOR CAUSE OF DEATH in pregnant women; any bleeding during pregnancy or after child birth therefore must be regarded as an EMERGENCY!

C. IRON DEFICIENCY ANAEMIA is a common complication in Nigerian Pregnant women. So pregnancy supplements containing IRON must be taken except otherwise stated!
A supplement like Pregnacare must be "supported" with Iron tablets (commonly called FERSOLATE) because the Iron quantity is not targeted for Nigerians who are more predisposed to Iron Deficiency Anaemia.

D. PRE-ECLAMPSIA AND ECLAMPSIA (hypertension/ high blood pressure in pregnancy) can be very fatal too!

E. HIGH PERFORMANCE LIQUID CHROMATOGRAPHY is the most accurate and sensitive test to detect genotype incompatibility. Only a few healthcare facilities in Nigeria have the machine to carry out this investigation.

It'd be wise to save your unborn child from the pains of SICKLE CELL by carrying out this investigation (AS vs AA vs SS).

F. RHESUS INCOMPATIBILITY also can cause abortion of a second baby and subsequent ones; when the "grandmother" theory plays out, the first baby can be affected too!

G. AMNIOCENTESIS can help your doctor detect birth malformations early; subsequent termination will be planned earlier too if the risks outweigh the benefits of keeping the baby.

(Down's syndrome, Turner's Syndrome, Klinefelter's syndrome etc have greater risks and disadvantages both on the child and care givers. Some of these come with intellectual disabilities)

H. WOMEN ABOVE 35 YEARS stand a higher risk of having children with birth malformations; as a man or a woman advances in age, this risk increases!

I. X-RAYS AND CT SCANS (the latter especially) must be avoided during pregnancy except the benefits far outweigh the risks.

J. Certain ANTIHYPERTENSIVE medications must be stopped if you are on them.

K. ANTI-SEIZURE drugs that hamper folic acid metabolism must be stopped 3 months before pregnancy too.

L. AMINOGLYCOSIDES such as GENTAMICIN have the capacity to cause defects in the ears and the kidneys of a child if taken during pregnancy.

M. SMOKING, DRINKING, DRUG/SUBSTANCE ABUSE during pregnancy have a highly negative impact on the baby you carry.

N. A CHAPERONE is an assistant that makes sure that a doctor does not sexually assault or molest you. Make sure you ask for a CHAPERONE. You are entitled to one. Chaperones are needed during doctor's examination and investigation processes because of possible medicolegal or litigation purposes. Pregnancy, delivery and postpartum period requires that you be examined & investigated ; you'll be in the labour room or theatre too. So chaperones are compulsory during these period!

O. FORCEPS DELIVERY of your child by a QUACK destroys the ability of your child's lower jaw bone to grow.

P. TETRACYCLINE causes severe and grossly shameful TOOTH DISCOLORATION in children less than 8years; whether administered to the child when they're in the womb or after birth.

Q. SWALLOWING TOOTHPASTE by an under-8 years has the capacity to cause similar TOOTH DISCOLORATION.

R. THE COLOSTRUM which is the first breast milk you produce after childbirth must not be discarded. This is the most important milk you will ever give your child because of the inherent immunity building capacity.

S. BREAST MILK ALONE must be given to the child for the first 6 months; appropriate foods can supplement this for the following 18 months.

T. The ANTERIOR FONTANELLE (the soft part of your baby's head) directly leads into the brain. Therefore, do not allow just anybody to carry your child to prevent BRAIN INJURY.

U. The BONES IN THE JOINTS of your growing child are responsible for elongation of bones and the consequent height of your child. INJURY right in any of these joints may lead to the child's inability to increase in height on both legs or one leg.

V. You have the capacity as a mother to determine HOW INTELLIGENT YOUR CHILD can be by giving him the right diet(breastmilk inclusive).

W. YOUR CHILD'S BRAIN is a Tabular Rasa (a clean sheet where you can write out exactly what you want your child to become). When you are deliberate about this, they can be icons like Ben Carson, Bill Gates and many more.

FINANCIAL BONUSES

FULFILLMENT OF MY PROMISES MADE WHEN MARKETING MY BOOKS

1. You will LEARN MY SECRET and invaluable lessons; learnt from the costly mistakes I made in attempts to invest money with other people and trade cryptocurrency on my own!

A. Do not give anyone, (whosoever) your money to trade forex or cryptocurrency (futures or derivatives) for you.

B. Always set "STOP LOSS" no matter how sure you are about the success of the trade.

C. Do not put all your eggs in the basket of cryptocurrency trading, forex trading or any other investments or businesses.

D. Always set TAKE PROFIT at any slightest profit you make. It is the profit you take from the cryptocurrency or forex market that becomes your own!

E. Learn cryptocurrency trading and Forex trading aggressively before any attempt to take trades on your own.

Cryptocurrency trading skills are one of the highest paid digital skills in the world!

A highly recommended teacher from whom I have learnt aggressively is Jackto Precious.

You can access his simplified, extremely detailed and exhaustive video course through the link below:

https://selar.co/p/ejtf?affiliate=yru1

https://selar.co/p/ejtf?affiliate=yru1

https://selar.co/p/ejtf?affiliate=yru1

Because this course has an exceedingly HIGH RETURN ON INVESTMENT, it is presently selling crazily. You can sell it too to other people with very limited resistance.

Here's the link:

https://selar.co/p/ejtf?affiliate=yru1

2. The SECRET REASON WHY I lost 700k to cryptocurrency trading in just one night and How I was able to recover from this loss within a space of 1 year!

A. I lost 700,000 naira in one night because I refused to set "STOP LOSS" at a reasonable point. 75 % of my funds were lost because I set my "stop loss" at a place where the market would have gone 75% south of the entry price.

B. I recovered in 1 year and still made triple the money I lost because I took a break from trading and focused on other areas that can bring in money for me.

Examples include:

i. Sales of my books: "SHINING THROUGH THE DARK TUNNEL",

https://selar.co/a1lj

and "SICKLE CELL UNMASKED".

https://selar.co/ve8u

ii. Aggressive marketing of our events management business and my sister's Instagram events management page.

Here's my sister's page:

https://www.instagram.com/atc.events/

respectively.

You can check out our works on the Instagram account and PATRONISE US NOW.

iii. BY SELLING OTHER PEOPLE'S HOTTEST READY-MADE COURSES:

I was forced to learn rapidly that I can make a massive income by selling READY MADE COURSES that talk about LEAVING NIGERIA for a greener pasture in CANADA.

These courses sell crazily because most people in Nigeria want to leave the country because of the sad financial set back, insecurity etc, that the country gave to them.

You can also benefit from these courses(BY STUDYING THE COURSE) if you have a dream to travel outside Nigeria.

Here are the links:

https://app.expertnaire.com/product/7595648168/7426540612

https://app.expertnaire.com/product/7595648168/7426540612?p=1

I STRONGLY RECOMMEND the first one!

You can also benefit from it by simply selling the course as an affiliate.

Here are the links:

https://app.expertnaire.com/product/7595648168/7426540612

https://app.expertnaire.com/product/7595648168/7426540612?p=1

I STRONGLY RECOMMEND the first one!

This very first course is a "3-STEP UNFAIR ADVANTAGE" any serious person can follow to relocate to Canada IN JUST MONTHS if you are really passionate about moving.

And YOU CAN ALSO MOVE YOUR ENTIRE IMMEDIATE FAMILY ALONG WITH YOU.

REGARDLESS OF YOUR AGE.
REGARDLESS of your education (the MINIMUM IS AN SSCE).

REGARDLESS of your MARITAL STATUS.

REGARDLESS OF IF YOU HAVE A FAMILY IN CANADA OR NOT.

The good part is that…:

YOU CAN ALSO SAVE AS MUCH AS 2 MILLION NAIRA IN THE PROCESS.

So, what are you waiting for? Click on this link; GET THE COURSE NOW AND BEGIN TO SELL TO OTHER PEOPLE!:

https://app.expertnaire.com/product/7595648168/7426540612

https://app.expertnaire.com/product/7595648168/7426540612?p=1

YOU CAN HAVE ACCESS TO EACH OF MY BOOKS, RESPECTIVELY, THROUGH THE LINKS ABOVE

3. All my SECRET knowledge about Marketing, Money Management and Investment, will also be LEAKED OUT TO YOU!

My main knowledge are found in the following books:

22 Immutable Laws Of Marketing by Trout and Al Ries and Jack Trout.

GET IT FOR FREE HERE:

https://www.pdfdrive.com/the-22-immutable-laws-of-marketing-figepgstaticnet-d17469280.html

30 Laws of Money by Dr. Abib Olamitoye.
GET THE BOOK HERE:

http://onehundredtenacademy.com/laws-of-money

How to Build a Business That Thrives in Your Absence by Dr. Abib Olamitoye.

GET THE BOOK HERE:

http://onehundredtenacademy.com/business-that-thrives

What I Want My Child To Know About Building a Great Life by Dr. Abib Olamitoye.

GET THE BOOK HERE:

http://onehundredtenacademy.com/Building-a-Great-life

For Copywriting, please kindly send me a Direct Message:

https://wa.me/2348020878841

You can also message me directly for an overview (SUMMARY) of the above courses and books:

www.ingramcontent.com/pod-product-compliance
Lightning Source LLC
Chambersburg PA
CBHW052159220526
45471CB00004B/1734